HOW WE SAID GOODNIGHT

Bardolf & Company

HOW WE SAID GOODNIGHT

ISBN 978-1-938842-00-9

Copyright ©2014 by Rachel Silsdorf

Published by Bardolf & Company
    5430 Colewood Pl.
    Sarasota, FL 34232
    941-232-0113
    www.bardolfandcompany.com

Cover design by Cathleen Shaw

How we said
Goodnight

Rachel Silsdorf

Bardolf & Company
Sarasota, Florida

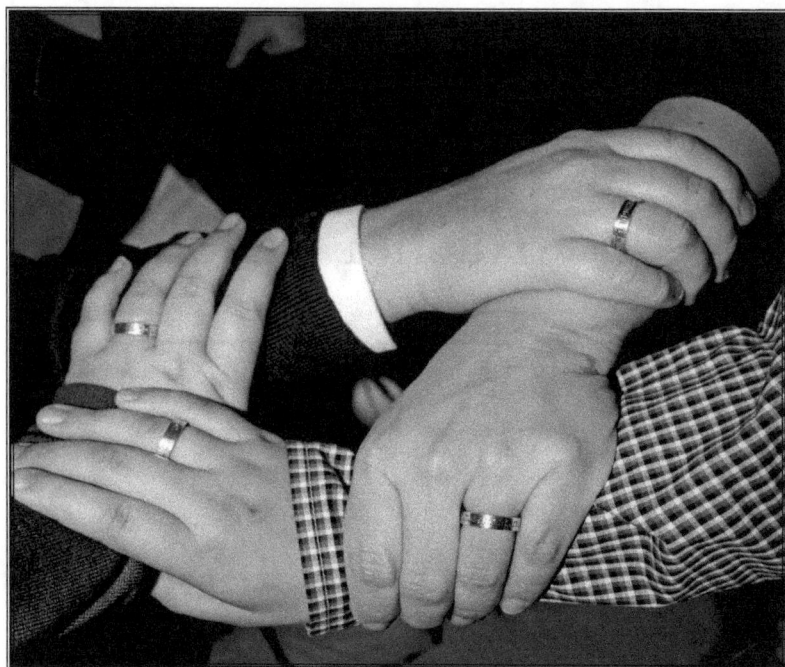

To my beautiful children
who remind me that life and love are verbs.

Emma

My heart started beating on the day of your birth.

Jonah

It found its rhythm on the day of yours.
You are my everything!

And always to

Arlan

the bravest person I have ever known.
Your epic humor, gentle kindness and wit
are a part of me. You're in my soul.
Marrying you was the single smartest decision
of my entire life.
Without you, without us, there is no me.
You are eternal, you live in me.

Contents

Acknowledgements

With profound appreciation to my family, particularly, Rebecca and Devon McArthur, Alex Ginsberg, Scott Silsdorf, Julie Silsdorf, and Renee Knight without whose constant love and support we would not be here today.

A very public thank you as well to the many friends and neighbors who sustained our household through Arlan's battle and since, including but certainly not limited to; Stephanie Murphy and Family, Rupali Desai and family, Jennifer Finn, Lisa and Marc Dopp, Mitch and Theresa Whealdon, Jennifer and Marty Ballard, Matt Francescon, and the Olde Sawmill community.

I would also like to express my thankfulness for the many kind and talented medical teams who cared for Arlan including Dr. Anterpreet Neki and team, Dr. Joel Mayerson and team, Dr. James Elder and team, Michelle Angelis, Chad and the many nurses and patient assistants who provided compassionate and capable care.

And finally, with deep gratitude to my dear friend Toni Teague who would not let me forget that the world was waiting to hear my words and to Ron Williams whose gentle love and support has sustained me.

Last, but certainly not least, my sincere gratitude to Chris Angermann of Bardolf & Company, who patiently edited my work and shepherded me through this process. Without you, Chris, this book would not have happened!

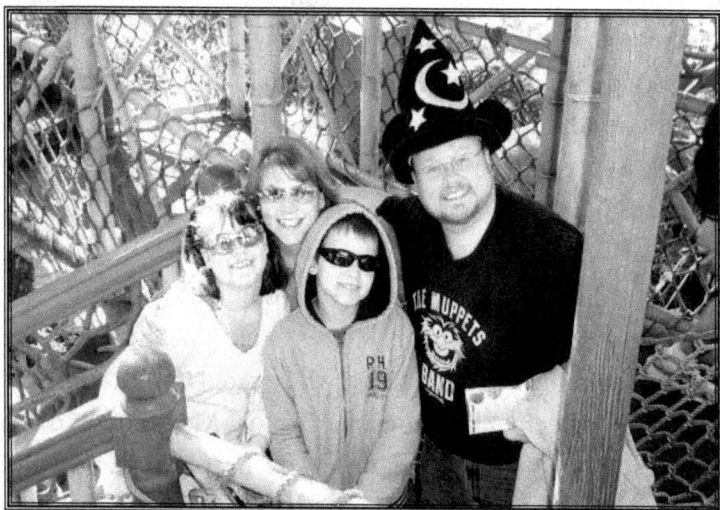

Emma, me, Jonah and Arlan
at an adventure park.

Prologue

I was unbelievably lucky, more so, in fact, than I even realized. My husband Arlan and I were basically decent kids who grew into reasonably mature adults. By the time we met in our late twenties, neither of us had led perfect lives, although Arlan was the epitome of responsible choices. We finished high school, went to college, graduated without major incident and got decent jobs. We had two beautiful children, Emma and Jonah, and lived a good, comfortable, middle-class existence. We were just not the sort of folks that bad things happen to. Although we faced some minor obstacles, most of the notable challenges were on the periphery of our lives and involved us lending support to siblings, friends or other family. We were people who made casseroles for others; who willingly watched their kids while they dealt with their crises.

So when Arlan was diagnosed with cancer in the spring of 2010, we were as unprepared as we could be.

There are three sides to every story – yours, mine and the truth, which likely lies somewhere in the middle. This book represents my version of truth. It is the story of my perception of what happened to my husband Arlan and my experience of caring for him through his journey with cancer. We often struggled and although for the most part we were very lucky to work with outstanding medical teams, whose kindness, care and compassion still humbles me, he did not always receive what I would consider exemplary medical care. That being said, I want to be clear that my intention in sharing our story is not to embarrass anyone unduly or diminish anyone's contribution. I do believe, however, that professionals carry an extra burden and responsibility to do their best, and there are lessons to be learned from Arlan's experiences for other cancer patients, their caregivers and yes, their medical staff.

I confess that I have always been a book hound. Before the days of the e-reader I could generally be found with stacks in my office, car and house, and so my natural inclination when we received the diagnosis was to get a book for caregivers. I found lots of books written by cancer patients and books about cancer in general, but none at that time specifically for caregivers that talked in frank terms about the experience; so that's what this is.

I kept an online blog throughout Arlan's journey. Based on that blog and my often painful, but treasured memories, I offer you whatever comfort and courage that, looking back on the experience of caregiving can suggest. I do not pretend to be an expert on cancer; there are doctors for that. I do not pretend to be an expert on caregiving or emotional trauma either; again there are psychologists, social workers and other professionals to help you with your own circumstances. What I am an expert on was how I cared for Arlan, and what I have learned from the experience to date, as that is an on-going journey. Our story is deeply personal, but not really unique. I will do my best to share with you what happened in the expectation that it may help you feel less alone in your own care giving journey.

Perhaps the most important lesson I learned was about hope, the many faces it takes and the way it evolves. Hope, my friends, is everlasting.

1

A Pain in the Leg

It all started innocently enough. We were preparing for Passover and I asked Arlan, "Can you grab the folding table from the basement?"

Passover is my favorite holiday, a time of family, laughter and some of our favorite foods. Being Jewish has always been more of a heritage than a religion in our house and Passover, for me, is Judaism at its best. Arlan, my husband of 14 years, had never been a lazy guy. While he was generally unmotivated to do projects around the house that I wanted completed, he was always helpful and pitched in with a smile.

He came up the stairs to set up the table, and I noticed again the limp that had been plaguing him for several months.

"Leg still hurting?" I asked.

"Yeah, guess I need to ice it again."

"Do me a favor and go make an appointment to have it looked at while I'm thinking about it"

This was met with a rolling of eyes and muttering under his breath, "Why do I have to do it while you're thinking of it?"

"Because you NEVER think of it," I answered loudly with more nastiness than necessary.

Again, rolling of eyes, followed by heavy sighing. I felt like a nagging wife, but he had been babying this leg for a long time. In the beginning of our marriage, he did not mutter under his breath and I was not a nagger, but as the years passed, we had become much more careless with each other, as couples inevitably do. We always joked that eventually we would end up like one of those little old couples you see in coffee shops, sitting at a table and never speaking to each other.

A few years ago Arlan took up running. One of his most charming and sometimes infuriating traits was his propensity to become completely engrossed in a hobby. He would learn every facet of what captivated his interest and amaze and, yes, frequently bore me with the depth of his knowledge of the obscure. He could do anything he set his mind to and when he decided to run a half marathon, despite being ridiculously out of shape, he approached it with his characteristic obsessiveness. He downloaded a training program for his iPod, did extensive research on-line and hooked up with a neighbor who ran and agreed to coach him. Sure enough, Arlan ran three half marathons before slipping off a curb in icy weather and spraining an ankle. By the time it healed, he had kind of left running behind and moved onto his next obsession.

During the summer of 2009, Arlan had discussed taking up running again and even gone out for a few short jaunts, but came back complaining of tightness in his right thigh. He iced it and we both assumed he had pulled something. Over Christmas that year Arlan took our kids, Jonah and Emma, then nine and 11, to visit his Christian family in Pennsylvania. He came home with a visible limp, complaining of pain in his thigh. He told me that one of our nieces had flopped down in his lap and that he had been in pain and limping ever since. I became concerned because the niece was not really big enough to have caused any real pain or damage to a man his size. I insisted he go to see his doctor.

He did so about a week later, came home and smugly reported, "It's nothing, just muscular. They gave me some exercises and said to ice it."

"Did they take an x-ray?"

"Nah, didn't need one."

"You should have insisted."

"If it doesn't go away on its own, they will."

"Did you tell them you were limping, that the pain keeps you up at night?"

"Yes, if it doesn't go away, I'll have an x-ray. Let it go."

On and off, I noticed Arlan limping and icing the leg. I did suggest quite a few times that he go back and have the x-ray, but when the leg seemed to be bothering him less, I didn't press the issue.

A few weeks later, his mother's fiancée died suddenly. She had been in the process of moving in with him and had stored many items at his home. Arlan's brother, Scott was overseas and could not help. His sister, Carla was fighting brain cancer and in the process of a divorce, so she would not be able to offer assistance either.

"Arlan, you have to go be with your Mom."

"I don't know, I'm so tired."

"She's your mother, you have to," I insisted. "She needs you."

Arlan packed the car and headed off. Less than a week later, he came back, looking pale and shaken. He was limping. I asked what happened and he said his leg was acting up. After moving his mom's things he was in so much pain he almost couldn't drive home. He had to stop a few times and walk around. I was alarmed and again begged him to have the x-rays. He iced the leg instead, and it improved again.

So finally in March when he was limping once again, I had had enough. "Make the appointment and don't come home without a fucking x-ray!"

"It's my leg, why are you so worked up?"

"Because you are clearly not adult enough to recognize you need help."

We had a huge fight, which finally ended in his making an appointment. I didn't really think much about it again; we went on that evening and had our usual jovial Passover holiday. Our table was full of family. We laughed and drank wine, sang and made the same tired jokes we make every year. The next day was back to life as usual. The kids were at school, Arlan and I worked. He continued to manage the kids before and after school, juggling their various activities. In many ways that I never took the time to notice our life was relatively ideal.

In retrospect, I wish we had paid more attention. Pain is a body's way of telling you something's wrong, and it would have been better for Arlan to listen sooner rather than ignore it and wait for it to go away.

2

Hurry up and Wait

The following week I was sitting in my office planning for summer, which was my busiest season as Director of Resident Services for a low income housing provider when my phone rang. "Hi honey, what's up?"

"Remember that doctor's appointment?"

His voice sounded shaky and suddenly my stomach was in my throat.

"I just finished. They ran the x-ray, and they found a tumor."

My mouth went dry. Before then, I didn't know that that was more than an expression, but a phenomenon I could actually experience. On the drive to our house, I was shaking when I called Arlan to assure him I was in the car.

"They don't know what kind of tumor it is," he told me. "I have to have an MRI tonight and a CAT scan.

"Okay, just hang on, I'm coming!"

I can't remember who all I called along the way – my sister? My mother? My mind was racing and I had a distinct feeling that something monumental was happening. I pulled into the garage and was out of the car before I had taken the key from the ignition. I ran through the door and into Arlan's expectant arms. I held him and thought, "Wait, it must be okay," his arms felt so solid around me.

The kids came home from school surprised to see me at such an early hour. After dinner, we made an excuse and headed out for his scans. We were quiet during the short drive to the testing center which is right next door to his doctor's office. What was there really to say? We arrived at the center and were the only ones there. It was dark outside already and although it was early April, still fairly cool. They took him into the imaging rooms immediately. I sat in the waiting room and thought about Arlan's mom, adjusting to the recent death of her fiancée, a man she had met and fallen for after eight years of widowhood, and I prayed that I would not regret my failure to insist that he get the x-ray on his return from helping her.

After we got home, we went to bed, but about three that morning, Arlan whispered "I'm scared."

"Me too, I didn't know you were awake."

"Can't sleep."

"Me either."

We lay there side by side in the dark waiting for morning to come. At some point I fell asleep briefly because I was woken by the alarm at 5:45. We showered, dressed, got the kids off and then drove to his doctor's office to have Arlan's blood drawn. While Arlan checked in, I went to the window to ask if we could wait after the lab work for the results to come in. The receptionist clicked away at her computer and informed me the results came in at 8:30 in the morning, but that the doctor had yet to see them.

"Please," I begged. "It's been a long night and we're scared."

She smiled kindly and explained that the doctor was booked and would call with results as soon as he could.

We left the office with heavy hearts and decided to have an early lunch. Surely, we reasoned, by the time we finished, the call would come and I would be free to head off to work. We chose a restaurant closer to downtown than usual so I could be nearer to my job. During the meal, Arlan's cell phone sat ominously on the table, an uninvited third guest intruding on our time. It never rang. We lingered over lunch as long as possible, and eventually decided we should go walk around Target and pick up some things we needed.

I hugged him as I got into my car – we had taken separate cars so I could go directly to work. "See you over there, let me know if he calls."

My heart beat so hard during the ride. I kept saying to myself, "I just know it's going to be okay, I have a good feeling." I pulled in at Target and looked around for Arlan. He was standing near the car waiting for me to get out.

When I did he simply said, "They called. It's cancer."

My head spun and in what in the months ahead would become a very familiar sensation I felt like I was watching this happening instead of experiencing it. "So, I said, "now what?"

"Let them have the leg. I don't care."

"Agreed. Whatever we have to do, it'll be okay."

"Yeah. Hey, we still need paper towels, let's go ahead into Target."

Inside, we pushed a cart around for a bit in silence. Neither of us touched anything on the shelves. Finally we decided to go home.

"Love you," Arlan said and kissed my lips softly before closing me safely in my car.

Once back at the house we sat across from each other at the kitchen table. The doctor's office called again and told Arlan he was scheduled to see a specialist at the local cancer hospital the following Tuesday for a biopsy. The kids came home from school and my daughter who had just turned 12, always clever for her age, immediately wanted to know what I was doing home two afternoons in a row.

Arlan and I looked at each other, and I said very matter-of-factly, "Well, you know how Daddy's leg has been hurting? He's sick and we are trying to figure out how to make it better."

"What's wrong with you Daddy?" she asked suspiciously.

Having worked in social services with kids for many years, I knew in theory that it was best to be honest, but say as little as possible. Calmly I said, "Well, he had an x-ray and some tests yesterday and he has cancer in his bone. Right now that's all we know."

Her eyes got huge. "Is that really bad?" she asked.

"Right now all we know is that it's there, but he looks fine to me."

Arlan smiled at her. "Don't worry Pookie Dookie. I'm going to a doctor to get this taken care of next week."

"We'll know more then and we promise not to keep secrets from you." I added.

Seemingly reassured, she got out her homework and Arlan and I each took a deep breath: hurtle one conquered. Fortunately, our nine year old was considerably more oblivious. Diagnosed with Asperger's Syndrome, Jonah was not one to notice much beyond his own nose. Even when something was brought specifically to his attention, he rarely discussed it much, despite being a deep thinker.

Arlan and I couldn't talk; couldn't even look at each other. The only thing we knew to do was to maintain our routine. As soon as the kids were in bed, we retreated to our separate computers. I began what would be an eight-month quest for information on mine. I googled "cancer bone tumor" and began to read. Some of the results were terrifying, some not too bad. After reading briefly,

I began to wonder if the cancer was originating in the bone. It seemed that most bone cancers occurred in the young or the elderly. The more I read, the more questions I had. Although frightened, by the time I logged off that night I had fairly well convinced myself that because of Arlan's age, the cancer was originating elsewhere. At some point we went to bed and spent another sleepless quiet night; together, but alone with our fear.

I headed to work the next day. This was a time of year when I really needed to focus, but it quickly became clear to me that that wouldn't be happening. Fortunately, as the director of the department I reported to the CEO, who could not have been more supportive or kind. Amy was not only my boss, but also someone who had become a mentor and friend. I made the decision to share what was going on with her right away so I would be in a position to do whatever was necessary without jeopardizing the program I was devoted to.

As the week progressed, we struggled to act normally. The specialist's office called and told Arlan to walk with crutches which he picked up the following day. They also told us that the suspected type of cancer was called an osteosarcoma. We separately read up on it, stunned by the rarity of it in adults his age.

3

Diagnosis

As we were driving to the hospital for his appointment, Arlan casually turned to me and said "You know, I meant to tell you something." This was followed by what felt like a very long pause, before he suddenly blurted out, "I've been coughing up blood."

"WHAT? How could you forget to tell me something like that? For how long?"

"I dunno, just a little bit, not that long. It didn't seem like a big deal. It might not even be related."

After that revelation, walking into the cancer hospital seemed a little surreal. Following a short wait, we were ushered into an examining room. A nurse came in and asked about a million questions, taking what was easily the most thorough medical history I had ever witnessed. We struggled to recall specific dates of various things, and before we knew it the doctor came in. He was about our age and similar in size and build to Arlan. His accent and manner indicated he was likely either a Midwest native or had lived in the area for a long time. He introduced himself as Dr. Mayerson, an orthopedic oncologist who specializes in bone cancers. Pulling out a copy of the X-rays taken the previous week, he showed us how the bone looked spongy, almost as if it had moth holes in it, and stated that it looked pretty convincingly like an osteosarcoma, although the diagnosis could only be confirmed with a biopsy.

A pathologist would do a fine needle biopsy right then and there, and the doctor would be able to tell us more before we left that day. The procedure would be uncomfortable, but only for a few minutes, and yield the quickest results. Arlan was already in considerable pain, so I requested he be given something to address his discomfort. Dr. Mayerson had a nurse get a pain pill to relieve the pain and take the edge off the biopsy.

Then the pathologist came in with a resident. He looked at the X-rays, asked some questions and got ready to start. Taking out a very long thin needle, he explained that he would be going in all the way to the bone in four spots on Arlan's thigh. Arlan was visibly shaken. I approached the bed, linked our hands together and leaned over him so he could only see me and nothing else. The pathologist inserted the needle and Arlan flinched and held his breath. I encouraged him to breathe as I stared deeply into his eyes and he sucked air between his teeth. After the pathologist had done the first three samples, the resident approached the bed and began the last series. Arlan broke out into a sweat and squeezed my hands, pumping them up and down. As the final needle was withdrawn from his leg, he began to shudder, crying like a small child, "It hurts." I gathered him against me like he was our son and could feel the tremors wracking his body. It took him about 10 minutes to calm down and recover from the cruel pain of the procedure. I was terrified, never having seen him react much to pain before. I spoke softly to him, calmingly reassuring him, although I was shaking inside.

In what felt like an unbelievably short time, Dr. Mayerson returned and in a rather serious tone, told us that it was indeed an osteosarcoma. I questioned this as my research had indicated it was so rare in adults our age. The doctor confirmed this and told us that the chances of developing an osteosarcoma at Arlan's age were about 1 in 30 million.

I cuffed Arlan's arm and said, "Why couldn't you have played the lotto?"

The doctor explained that it was not genetic, but just something that happens sometimes. Our next steps would be to have an MRI, CAT scan and PET scan, which would allow them to stage his tumor and provide us with more information in order to form a treatment plan. Using the crutches was necessary as breaking the leg could be catastrophic because it would release the active cancer trapped in the bone into the bloodstream.

We sat there stunned, struggling with what to say.

"So my kids are safe; they won't get this?" was Arlan's first question.

Dr. Mayerson reiterated that there is no known genetic link.

I rolled the word "osteosarcoma" around in my head and asked, "What's the bottom line? What will it take to beat this?" I've always been a bottom line kind of person. Just tell me how bad it is, how long the fight would be—I never doubted that we could beat it.

"Just take the leg," I insisted. "It's okay. We can work around this."

The doctor patiently explained that he was a surgeon and when the time came, he would perform the operation. But for now, he would be turning us over to Doctor Neki, an oncologist who specialized in concocting the right chemotherapy cocktail. He assured us that his colleague was an excellent doctor and eventually brought him in to meet us.

The oncologist was a tall, bulky gentleman. His twisted beard, turban and accent suggested he was of Indian descent. He also conveyed the aggressive nature of this type of cancer and wanted to get started with chemotherapy as soon as possible. He would do a few rounds and then reevaluate if, perhaps, Arlan was ready for surgery. He would schedule follow-up tests for later that week, as well as a power port placement to dispense the chemicals.

Before we left, Dr. Neki asked if we had children. I felt as if the air had been sucked from the room, and my mouth tasted of bile. Arlan's eyes were wide as he nodded.

"Are you planning to have more?" the doctor asked.

Arlan half shook his head and half shrugged.

A pin drop would have echoed like a heavy bolt in the room as Dr. Neki explained that he was asking only because the chemo would likely leave Arlan sterile after the first round, and if we wanted more children, we should make an emergency appointment to immediately freeze some of his sperm. Arlan and I both began to breathe again as the panic passed and we realized that the oncologist was not about to deliver scary news implicating a genetic link to our children.

As we were about to leave, I remembered how tricky it was for Arlan to navigate parking lots with his new crutches, especially in the rain, and asked about a handicap placard. My mind was racing with all sorts of questions and I started to make silent lists of things that needed to be done, but I smiled with what I hoped was unruffled confidence and took all the various papers we'd been given.

On the way home, we drove in silence. Neither of us could find words, and even had I had some, I don't know if I could have gotten them past the lump in my throat. Finally, Arlan suggested we should try to eat something. I nodded and shrugged helplessly when he asked where we should go. Eventually, I called my sister Rebecca, who had been waiting by the phone for news. We met her and my brother- in-law, Devon, at a small restaurant. Arlan and I poked at our food. With the lump in my throat still there, I was unable to swallow as we relayed the details of our hospital visit.

Arlan smiled optimistically setting the tone we would take for the entire battle. "This is going to be a bitch," he said, "but what choice do I have? I gotta beat it."

I nodded my head emphatically. "Whatever we have to do," I assured him, "we're in this together."

He squeezed my hand and looked at Devon conspiratorially. "Already off work today, may as well check out Micro Center," he said with a grin.

Arlan was the quintessential geek. He loved all things technical, could fix or build anything and simply adored time spent strolling through the electronic store. Fortunately, my brother-in-law shared this affinity for technology and the two of them took off.

In the darkest times of our lives, my older sister and I have always held each other up. We can frequently go weeks or longer without speaking, but I know there is nothing she won't do for me, and vice versa. Although Rebecca is an amazing woman, she has had her share of struggles. With four children and on her third marriage, she often leaned on me and Arlan for various forms of support.

That day, Rebecca and I sat silently in the booth after the boys left. I looked up and saw a tear trickling down her face, and as if a dam broke, I let go and collapsed into sobs. Rebecca came around to my side, and I felt her begin to rock me gently. I don't know how long I cried in her arms, but eventually, I stopped.

I blew my nose and said, "That's enough. I have to get this together."

We looked at each other, and Rebecca said, "We're with you."

I nodded and we walked out of the restaurant.

4

Testing and Telling

That week was a jumble of medical tests. They wanted to set his "baseline" to help them chart Arlan's progress and recognize how best to treat the disease. We wandered through the endless maze of hallways of the two other hospitals connected to the cancer center. We sat in one waiting room after another. I learned to work on my laptop by setting up a mini office in a corner with coffee and my cell phone on a side table. I returned e-mails, wrote reports and continued my research while Arlan was poked, prodded, photographed and scanned from every angle, inside and out.

On non-testing days we made phone calls to the various family members that needed to be told. We agonized over telling Arlan's mom Julie the news. A widow for nine years, she was still grieving from the death of her fiancée. Meanwhile, she was also the full-time caregiver for Arlan's only sister, Carla, who was in the middle of a separation from her husband, had two young daughters and had been recently diagnosed with brain cancer. Additional stress and anguish came from the loss of Julie's youngest sister to stomach cancer only a few months after diagnosis. In light of these many burdens, we worried over how to tell her our scary news.

Arlan also had a brother, Scott, younger by two years, who was living on a naval base in Japan with his wife Beth and their two young daughters. Although Arlan had always expressed his adoration for Scott, I had never had the chance to get to know him well. Arlan called Scott to talk about his illness and I happened to answer the phone when he called back. Having had little or no relationship with Scott, I stumbled a little when I realized it was he and said, "Arlan's sick, hang on," and turned the phone over to Arlan. Because Scott lived so far away, he was not a viable option to help in telling their mom.

After a few days of worrying, I put a call in to Arlan's Aunt Rose. Arlan comes from a large, extended Pennsylvania Dutch family, and he adores all of his aunts and uncles, but Aunt Rose has always held a special place in his heart. She is one of those people who has the rare ability to make you feel special and loved just by the smile in her voice. Although I had never called her before in my fourteen years of marriage to her nephew, Aunt Rose answered as if we spoke daily and she was thrilled to hear from me.

When I explained what was going on and that we were afraid of how to tell Arlan's mom, she said, "Good girl, you did the right thing. Katie (Arlan's other surviving aunt) and I need to be with her when she hears this."

"Everything's okay" I assured her. "We have this under control and, really, Carla is way sicker."

"Maybe not," Aunt Rose replied, sending a chill of foreboding down my spine.

The next morning Aunt Rose called back to tell me they would be taking Mom to dinner that evening and that we should call at seven. She assured me that she and Katie were prepared to stay with her as long as they were needed and urged me to just focus on Arlan. At the appointed time, Arlan called his mother to break the news while I stood by in the doorway to his home office. As he dialed, Arlan turned his chair to face the wall. I saw his shoulders sag several times as the phone rang. His voice was small and subdued as he greeted his mother. He began to talk, and then turned toward me. Looking young and helpless, he held out the phone to me. I could see his mouth opening, but no words were coming.

Taking a deep breath, I took the receiver and said, "Mom, I need to tell you that they found cancer in Arlan's leg. It's an osteosarcoma. We are in the process of having it staged."

Arlan had been crying silently and drying his tears he reached for the phone again. I asked if I should pick up an extension and he nodded gratefully. I ran upstairs to our room and picked up in time to hear him explain that he WAS going to beat this. She agreed and talked about the importance of maintaining a positive attitude. Over and over she apologized that she couldn't come right away because of Carla and her girls. Arlan assured her that we were okay and I promised to stay in close touch.

We hung up and I heard Arlan on the stairs. He came into the bedroom and lay next to me on the bed, resting his head against my chest, and again, I held him like a child as he cried silently.

5

Preparing for Treatment

Early one morning we reported to the hospital for port placement. Although this is a minor procedure, it required a visit to the OR. After going through the admissions process for the third time that week, we were ushered into a room where a nurse ran an IV. Arlan has always struggled when having IVs placed or blood drawn, often needing several tries to hit a vein, but in his usual calm and stoic manner, he accepted her poking around in his arm.

Grinning at me he said, "Well, the good news is that after today they can just use the port, no more arm pricks."

"There is that" I replied optimistically.

The nurse explained that Arlan would be getting something called a dual power port which she professed to be "awesome" as it would provide two separate lines at once. Because Arlan was facing a really aggressive cancer, he would be getting very aggressive chemotherapy, which meant multiple types of chemo going simultaneously that could not be mixed outside the body. Also having the dual power port would allow blood to be drawn even as IV drips were going.

Apparently, chemo patients needed to receive blood or blood products frequently to increase their white cell count to help fight infection. All these things, the nurse assured us, would be eased through the placement of this port. She showed us the small plastic Y-shaped device with bumps and explained that the tubes coming off the two prongs would provide direct access to Arlan's bloodstream.

However tedious and exhausting our many appointments were, I can never adequately express how empowering and helpful it was to have medical staff take this kind of time with us. This nurse, while undoubtedly busy, acted as if she had nothing more important to do than equip us with knowledge about the procedure and why it was necessary. Armed with information, we felt confident and reassured.

Eventually, Arlan was moved to a large room with lots of bays separated by curtains. His admission bracelet was checked once again, and his IV hung in the new location. I perched on the stool next to his bed, while he smiled up at me nervously. A young man and woman, dressed in surgical uniforms from cap to foot covers, danced past our bay, loudly joking with each other about what they had done the night before. Arlan became visibly tense as their carrying on became more intrusive. When his nurse returned to check on him, he asked who they were and she explained that they transported patients to the OR suites and assisted during the procedures. When she saw Arlan's eyes grow large, she quickly assured him that he was simply having a port placed and another member of the surgical team would be doing his procedure in short order. She asked if he brought his C-pap, the machine he uses at night to protect his breathing because of sleep apnea. He hadn't, since we didn't know he would need it.

Shortly thereafter, an attendant came over and explained he would be setting up a C-pap for Arlan. He approached the bed and began to unwrap a mouthpiece. Having read much about the danger of infection for cancer patients, I asked if he had washed his hands. He rolled his eyes and said in a controlled calm voice that he washed his hands all day. Then he strutted over to the hand sanitizer, rubbed some lotion into his hands and held them up to me. Although I apologized and explained that I was nervous after everything I had read, he reminded us that none of this would be necessary if we had brought Arlan's C-pap from home.

After he left, an older doctor approached and said he would be inserting the port. Arlan appeared calmed by his professional manner. The doctor told me to go to the family waiting area and check in so they could notify me when Arlan was in recovery. I kissed my husband. Before I left, I was given a tracking number and told that the procedure would take about a half hour or so.

I entered the family waiting area, juggling my purse, laptop bag, Arlan's backpack with his netbook, magazines and other papers, his crutches and his bag containing his clothes, wallet and etc. Nervously I checked in with the volunteer, a kind older woman, who smiled sweetly, and wrote down my name and what color clothes I was wearing. She promised they would page me just as soon as Arlan was out of surgery and handed me a disc that would light up and buzz as if I were waiting for a table at a restaurant. As I walked away awkwardly carrying all of our loot, she called and asked if I would like to leave the crutches and other materials behind her desk. Thinking I would only be there for a very short time and nervous about losing something, I declined and parked myself in a nearby chair where I could watch the board with the tracking numbers.

I sat there with my mind racing and remembered my first date with Arlan as if it were yesterday. I was 24 and a little nervous about seeing someone I had never met before, although we had spoken on the phone several times. The date had been arranged by my older sister. We were going to join her and her boy-friend for dinner and then a movie. I opened my apartment door, and there he stood.

He had warm blue gray eyes and huge dimples and wore a goofy cowboy hat. He handed me a single red rose and introduced himself—from then on, he never appeared for a date without bringing a red rose. I felt almost immediately comfortable and invited him in. We sat in the living room, waiting for Rebecca and Gang to arrive. His eyes twinkled as he talked about the many places he had visited in his work as an electronic engineer, installing systems around the world. I remember liking the sound of his voice. The rest of the evening went well, too. At the end, we returned to my apartment and took my dog for a short walk, Arlan leaned in and kissed me and I remember thinking, I will marry this man.

In 1995, after trying for two years and undergoing multiple rounds of fertility drugs, I became pregnant with our first child. In the fall of that year, around the time I was 5 months pregnant, Arlan was laid off from his job. Although I had a great job myself, I was really worried, but Arlan remained calm.

"I'll get a job," he kept assuring me.

"When?" I would irritably reply.

"Working on it."

This pattern went on for a few weeks until I rushed home from work one late morning after a bout of the nausea that plagued me for most of the pregnancy. I needed to change my clothes. When I walked into the house and found Arlan sitting on the couch in his boxer shorts eating Captain Crunch and watching TV, I lost it. I yelled and carried on about how I was pregnant and working and he was doing nothing. I changed clothes and stomped out of the house. That afternoon Arlan attended a job fair and came home employed.

That was the thing about Arlan and me; everything always worked out for us. We struggled to get pregnant but we had two beautiful, bright, charming children—Emma who had just turned

12 and Jonah who was 9. They were our everything. He got laid off but found a job and was even able to work from home and provide before and after school care for the kids. Our marriage had been through its share of challenges, but we always landed on our feet.

These were the thoughts that I held onto as I sat in that waiting room, clutching the disc, waiting to hear I could take him home.

After about two hours, the board hadn't changed and I hadn't been paged. My cell phone rang. It was Arlan cheerfully asking what I was doing.

"Waiting to hear you're out of surgery."

He laughed and said he had been in a room for almost an hour and had just finished lunch.

"They never called or updated me," I explained.

"Sorry sweetie."

I found his room in another part of the hospital and couldn't help but smile as I came in and saw him flipping TV channels.

"You ready to go?" he asked with a grin.

I helped him dress while he explained that he had woken up from surgery downstairs and had repeatedly asked them to call me. When I didn't come, he eventually decided to try my cell. We laughed at the silliness of me sitting in the family waiting room surrounded by all our stuff.

As we left the hospital, he assured me that the port placement wasn't too bad. He mentioned that his chest felt a little tender but brushed it off as no big deal. He was just glad to be away from that pre-op room and the insensitive joking of the two staff members passing by.

Normally easy going and innately kind, he shook his head and said, "I get that people want to have fun at work, but I guess they don't realize how scary it is to be down there."

"Yeah, that was a bit creepy," I agreed and dodged his hands as he tried to take his backpack and my laptop bag despite being on crutches and having just come out of surgery.

Two days later we returned to the hospital for the final imaging. We had each done our homework, researching carefully and silently the various tests that were ordered and what results we should hope for, knowing that whatever the outcome, it would likely dictate much of our lives moving forward. I am not a religious person, my own lack of faith dwarfed only perhaps by Arlan, who not only found the belief in God and religion a waste of time but also illogical and somewhat annoying. But as they led him away to the imaging rooms, I prayed for all I was worth.

As we left the hospital that day, Arlan quietly said to me, "it's in my lungs."

"How do you know, what did they say?"

"Nothing. They didn't say anything, I just know."

6

The Stage is Set

Over the next five days life was as normal as possible. I began to make lists of things I needed to do. Knowing that Arlan would have no immune system left, the number one priority was getting the house cleaned and sanitized. I knew I was a crappy housekeeper with a home far messier than it should have been; but no worries, I called a cleaning service, a duct cleaner and carpet cleaner. Yes, Arlan's home office was a cluttered mess of years' worth of computer parts, hobby pieces, papers and miscellaneous junk that made it nearly impossible to walk through even if you weren't on crutches, but having recruited a small army of relatives and close friends it would all be getting set to right while he received his chemo.

My nephew Alex, then a college student, called me the day after the scans. I love all my nieces and nephews, but Alex has always held a special place in my heart. My sister, Rebecca, married early and started her family right away. Like many young marriages, it didn't last. By the time her kids were two and four, she was divorced and living in family housing at the local university while she finished her degree.

I was a graduate student living on the other side of a parking lot, literally a shopping center away. I helped her care for her four-year-old daughter, Sarah, and two-year-old son, Alex, and we all grew up together. Alex was a strong kid, bright and curious, but easily frustrated and quick to anger. I can still recall the feeling of his small body in my arms as I held him through a tantrum and listened to him sob. As he got older, we continued to be close, and he impressed me with his keen insights and dedication to those he loves. I wasn't surprised to hear from him.

He asked when Arlan would start treatment and said, casually, "I got you covered at the house."

When I asked him to repeat himself, he explained that he was planning to stay with my kids and dogs as much as needed. It brought tears to my eyes. I thanked him with a lump in my throat and hung up quickly.

I spoke to my mother during that time as well. She and her husband were scheduled to take a short cruise. I urged them to go, although she offered to cancel several times. I reminded her that there was nothing she could do to change what was going on and that at this point we knew very little. Arlan and I were scheduled to return to the oncologist the following Tuesday morning.

I was keeping up a good front, but the strain took its toll. Until then, even during the most stressful times of our marriage, we had always been able to connect through physical intimacy, but now we were intensely focused on what was to come. Although we held each other frequently, so great was our distraction that we did not even take the time to make love.

The night before the appointment, neither of us was able to sleep.

Around 3:30 in the morning, Arlan suddenly said, "I've been reading about bio-feedback"

"Really, like what?"

"I read about someone who imagined that the cancer in his body was like a Pac-Man game. I'm going to do that. I'm going to picture the little Pac-Man eating all the cancer cells. The Pac-Man can be the chemo, gobbling up all the bad cells as he goes."

At some point we gave up on trying to sleep. The first light of dawn had not yet reached the sky when we dragged ourselves out of bed. As I stood in front of the bathroom mirror checking my appearance before going to wake the children, Arlan wrapped his arms around my shoulders from behind. I reached up to cover his hands with my own, and briefly closed my eyes as I melted into his familiar and comforting warmth. I simply could not imagine that this was really happening; Arlan was the oxygen of my world.

Later in the hospital waiting room, we sat side by side, hand in hand, saying nothing, before being ushered into the exam room where Arlan took his seat on the table as I sat in a side chair. Ten minutes may have passed or an hour—time stretched and stood still. Eventually, Dr. Neki, the oncologist, came in. He sat down and asked Arlan about the pain and how he had been doing this week. Arlan responded with monosyllabic grunts, shrugs and nods. I sat on my hands to prevent what I really wanted to do – grab the doctor by the lapels of his white coat and demand he tell us immediately that all was well.

The physician's assistant came in and sat at the computer in the room to enter notes. As Dr. Neki began to speak, he began to sketch what looked like the outline of a human body on the scrap paper attached to his clipboard. Then he began to make dots in the chest area and my head dropped forward, chin to chest. My despair was so great that even the effort to hold my head up was too much. I knew in that moment that not only was the cancer in Arlan's lungs, it was all over them. Neither Arlan nor I spoke for several moments. I sat there with my head hanging, using my hair to shield my face.

Finally, Arlan said, "So this means lung surgery too?"

Dr. Neki explained that our next step would be to aggressively attack the cancer with chemotherapy and then reevaluate how things were going.

I found my voice, "So is this stage 4 then?"

Dr. Neki regarded me somberly. "Yes, stage 4, this is the worst, the worst it could be."

"But he can still beat it?"

"No, this is not beatable. We can try to hold things off as long as possible, maybe if things respond really well to chemo buy some time, but he cannot survive this."

Some part of me heard him say those words, but it was as if we were all under water. I took in the sounds, but the meaning of the words was unintelligible. I fought to take in breath; I stared at my shoes, at the closed door, anywhere but at Arlan knowing that I needed to rally my internal strength before I could face him. As my eyes danced around the room, my brain rearranged the doctor's words into something I could accept. We would beat this.

As the shock slowly receded, we began to ask for statistics and options. Dr. Neki explained that until we saw how Arlan responded to treatment, it was difficult to know. People could potentially live for many years with lung nodes; however, he was not optimistic that Arlan would be one of them because of the number of nodes. Above all, it was important to begin treatment quickly and aggressively. He wanted Arlan to be admitted tomorrow for the first round of chemo, which would be given on an in-patient basis for five days in a series of 24 hour drips.

We heard all his words, we did. And yet as he and his team filed out of the office, closing the door gently behind them to "give us a moment" Arlan and I looked at each other and silently agreed; Dr. Neki was mistaken. This was a winnable fight; Arlan would beat this, no doubt about it.

"This is gonna be tough," he said.

I agreed. "You're in for a miserable battle."

"We'll get through it."

"Absolutely!"

We stared at each other in stunned silence.

"What are we going to tell the kids?" he asked.

"The truth" I responded. "It's bad, not the results we hoped for, but we are going to find a way."

"Yeah," he said, "but I don't like this doctor—way too negative!"

"I agree, but the sooner we start fighting the better, let's give him a chance and see if he improves."

We wrapped our arms around each other, both drawing and offering warmth and support. As we had from the early days of our relationship, we anchored each other, squared our shoulders and then, heads held high, left the hospital.

One the way home, Arlan called his mom with an update.

I began to make calls as well, including my office to explain that Arlan would start chemo the next day and that I would be with him and unable to come into work for the rest of the week. Amy, my superior, was unwaveringly supportive and assured me that I could just take the time.

"Thank you," I responded, "but this is going to be a long haul, and I might as well get into the groove of working remotely now because I do not plan to leave him alone at the hospital."

Amy encouraged me to do what I needed to do.

By the time our children got home from school, we had made plans for Alex to arrive the next day, finished all the necessary calls to other relatives, informed the schools, and were ready to talk. They knew of course that we had seen the doctor and arrived looking for answers. Emma admitted that she had been unable to focus well at school.

Like most parents, my gut instinct has always been to shield my children from pain and the scary stuff, and this was no different.

First and foremost, I am Mom! By then, I had all but obliterated any remnants of the echo in my head of the doctor's negative prognosis; I was fully focused on cure.

Smiling reassuringly I sat the kids down with some sliced apples and explained. "Daddy's pretty sick; sicker than we originally thought."

Emma's eyes began to flood with tears, Jonah looked away.

With determination to comfort both my babies—and myself—I gently took hold of Jonah's chin and turned his face toward me. I smiled confidently, maintained eye contact with them each in turn, and said, "This is going to be a long and hard fight. This was not the news we had hoped for, but no matter how bad things are, Daddy is strong and young and we believe he will beat it. No matter what, we will be fine."

The kids cried softly for a few minutes. I alternately rubbed their backs and gave out hugs.

When they had calmed down, I said, "We have a lot to get done. Daddy starts chemo in the morning." I continued, "Do you know what chemo is? It stands for chemotherapy, which is a group of medicines they give in different combinations and different ways to fight cancer."

Emma made a face and explained to her brother "Chemo is like poisons they give you to kill cancer cells."

How and what this child knew constantly amazed me. Emma, walked, talked and read at a very early age. Not only has she always possessed an uncanny ability to absorb and retain information that is way beyond her years, she also, even as a young child, could empathize with everyone around her. Jonah, is much more stoic, the embodiment of the old adage that quiet rivers run deep. As his sister explained about the harmful dichotomy of chemo—the drugs destroy both cancer and beneficial cells, compromising the body's immune system—his eyes widened. He began swallowing rapidly and got up silently to withdraw to the basement where a TV with a game console provided a refuge.

Emma was capable of absorbing more information, so I explained what was in store for us: an aggressive, 5-day treatment in the hospital. I would be staying with Daddy at the hospital to help the nurses take care of him. I would make sure to see her and Jonah every day and call them all time. The chemo itself wouldn't be painful—he would be basically lying in a bed with tubes in him to give him the medicine—and she could call him and visit.

Arlan came into the kitchen and slung an arm around her as he sat down in the chair next to her. "You gonna visit me at the hospital Pookie Dookie?" he asked.

She immediately responded, "Yes."

Jonah opened the basement door, came up behind Arlan and hugged him tight. Jonah has always given the world's best hugs. He and Arlan shared a kinship that allowed them to understand one another without words. They were much alike in so many ways, Arlan often referred to Jonah as his "mini me." While I found myself at times helpless to comfort him, Arlan could generally find a way.

Reaching up and wrapping his own arm around Jonah's neck, he said, "Love you buddy."

Later that evening, I went on the computer to look up the two medications Arlan would receive in the morning. By then, he looked exhausted, but when I glanced at the clock and told the kids it was time to start getting ready for bed, he immediately got up.

"Relax," I told him, "I'll get them."

"No way," he immediately shot back. "I may not see them for five days, and who knows what condition I'll be in when I get back. I'm putting my kids to bed."

He had rarely spoken to me in such a sharp and serious tone. I turned back to the computer and he followed the kids upstairs.

When I was pregnant with Emma, my sister gave me a CD of lullabies so beautiful it made me weepy (when I was pregnant everything made me a little weepy). I played the music every night, with headphones against my stomach hoping that when she was finally born, we would be able to play the music for her and calm her. I have no idea if it worked, but we did the same thing for Jonah. After they were born, we put them in their cribs each night with the music softly playing. It became an important part of our bedtime routine for many years. At ages 9 and 12, our kids really no longer required lengthy bedtime routines, but Arlan and I had long cherished these quiet moments with them. Since Jonah's birth, he and I took turns reading to each child, me with Jonah one night while Arlan read to Emma, and then lying down with them for two songs. Then Arlan and I would switch rooms and stay for two more songs with the other child.

In this way we each got to spend a few one-on-one minutes with both Jonah and Emma every day. Not only did this give us time to hear the details of their day, talk about things that were on their minds and enjoy a little snuggle with each, but it also allowed us to go back downstairs and have time to ourselves, or with each other, without feeling that we were neglecting the kids. When one of us was really caught up with work, tired or sick, the other would read with both kids. In so many ways things in our home had been idyllic for so many years that the idea of anything truly interrupting that was inconceivable.

That night after Arlan followed the kids upstairs, I learned about the potential side effects of the chemo, feeling increasingly sick about what I was reading. I eventually shut the computer down and headed upstairs. As I neared the top, I could hear Arlan and the kids in our bedroom. I sank onto one of the steps and listened to them giggling. I could picture the three of them stretched out on our king size bed, Arlan in the middle, intermittently tickling each kid. I swallowed hard several times and fought back tears as I sat there eavesdropping on my family, desperately wanting to wrap them all in a protective embrace.

7

Chemo

Having had little sleep, we reported to the oncologist's office with taut nerves, but a good attitude. Arlan was ready to visualize the chemo killing the cancer Pac-Man-style, and I was hopeful. We must have been quite a sight as we lugged two laptops, a small rolling suitcase and a duffel bag around.

We started in phlebotomy where the technicians wanted to draw Arlan's blood. After they pushed around on his chest with their fingers to locate the port, I saw him flinch and heard him hiss as they finally inserted the needles. My heart broke a little more, but I took a deep breath and reminded myself that my role was to witness—if he could tolerate it, I could watch it. The nurse said that the area was sore because the port had so recently been placed and that it would be fine in no time. I smiled, reassured, and glad that needle pricks were one concern I could soon cross off my list. After Arlan had been carefully weighed and had the leg with the tumor examined, we were sent to admissions.

Check-in was both an easy and frustrating process. We gave our names, wrote a check for $200 and were told that amount would be due at each admission. Then we were shuffled to another area to wait for an open room. As we sat there, I couldn't help silently calculate the toll that the $200 checks would take on our savings account. Like many families, we basically lived paycheck to paycheck, but through careful planning and incredible good fortune we had managed to put a little away over the years for a rainy day. It didn't take an accountant to figure out that we were entering monsoon season and we were among the lucky households who could even write these checks. I deliberately chose not to think about what we would do when the money ran out. I didn't have the mental energy at that point.

The minutes turned into an hour, then two, before a kind receptionist handed us vouchers for the hospital cafeteria. Upon arrival, we were struck by two things: the unappetizing self-serve food choices and filthy appearance—there were left-over crumbs and trash everywhere. Ordinarily I would not have batted an eye, but knowing from my research into what it would take to protect Arlan from germs and especially food borne pathogens, which posed a particularly heinous threat to chemo patients, I was shocked.

In retrospect, I understand that the hospital has a tremendous number of details to attend to. Still, while this unsavory cafeteria provided more discomfort than actual danger, I think hospitals would be smart to remember that appearances go a long way toward inspiring or undermining the confidence of patients and their families. We picked at our lunches before returning to the waiting room for another two seemingly interminable hours.

Eventually we were called and taken up to Arlan's room, which to our surprise, turned out to be very small and semi-private. Another man—bald, sallow and emaciated—was sleeping in the bed by the window. As Arlan would be spending the next five days there, the lack of privacy was an immediate concern. I saw the look on his face, turned right around and went to the nurse's station. When I asked how we could get a private room, I was told there were none available and they would put him on a waiting list in case one opened up.

A jovial woman bustled in and introduced herself as Michelle, the physician's assistant. She explained that she would be in to see Arlan daily, coordinate his treatment during his hospital stay and be available to answer questions or convey our concerns to other staff. Looking at her open smile and gentle, compassionate face, I believed her. She examined Arlan's leg and looked at his port a couple of times. After consulting her clipboard, she told us that they had accessed the port using the wrong needles and they would have to be re-done. Needless to say, this was not happy news considering how uncomfortable it had been to access the port the first time. Gripping Arlan's shoulder consolingly, Michelle assured him that it would get much better.

When she breezed out of the room, I followed her into the hall and again pressed my concern about a private room. She smiled warmly and agreed that all patients facing this kind of aggressive treatment really ought to have their own room. That was why they were building a new hospital which would open in 2014, and have only private rooms. Since that would do Arlan no immediate good, she promised to check to see if anything would open imminently. As I watched Michelle bustling on to the next room, I wondered if I had made a friend into a foe. On the surface her cheery, straightforward demeanor was exactly what I needed in an ally, and I hoped that I would be able to grow this relationship.

Resigned to make the best of things, I began to take out some items I had packed to help Arlan stay focused and "warm" up his room a little. I placed them where he would see them as soon as his eyes opened—framed 8x10s of both kids and an absolutely adorable painting that Jonah had done in second grade of him and Arlan smiling from the windows of the monorail at Disney. In the picture they have the same smile and the same yarn hair; only with Jonah it's on top of his head and in Arlan's case, it's his beard.

I smiled confidently, telling him to keep his "eyes on the prize, baby." I thought that under the watchful gazes and bright smiles of our children, Arlan would be constantly reminded that what he was fighting for was a complete cure to enjoy our family fully again. Everyone who came into the room commented about how beautiful the children were and Arlan beamed with pride.

By five that afternoon, the ports had been re-accessed with the correct needles (painful but done), the first two bags of chemo hung, and an admission questionnaire reviewed. We were sitting quietly when the door opened and his roommate's visitors arrived. Cancer knows no bounds—rich, poor, black, white, sophisticated or simple, we all get sick. Arlan and I have always considered ourselves to be open- minded, accepting sort of people. Having worked as a Social Worker for nearly 20 years I had met my share of interesting folks, but I was ill prepared for who entered. When the room door opened, a woman who weighed easily 400 pounds wheeled in on a scooter. With her came another woman on foot, who was only slightly smaller.

They drove and waddled past us calling out loudly, "Hey, you awake? WAKE UP!"

Once seated on the other side of the curtain, they unceremoniously announced that their relative would need to go to a nursing home when he left the hospital as they were not picking up after his "nasty ass" and "risk getting AIDS." He responded that if he didn't get to come back home he was not giving them the social security checks, and anyway, he didn't have AIDS, only HIV.

This was the first of many increasingly bizarre encounters with family and friends that we would hear through the curtain. Often we tried to take Arlan's IV pole and go elsewhere. Although the roommate was clearly very sick, he did provide some macabre comic relief. One of the first things he would do when anyone came to visit was order a tray of food. Unlike most chemo patients who struggled to find any food palatable, let alone hospital fare, he would order multiple entrees and side dishes for each meal, explaining to each dietician that he wanted everything to be served soft, as he had no teeth. One afternoon while enjoying a visit with some friends, he lamented that he would like to have a burger from White Castle because they are so soft. This launched the trio into reminiscing about when they all worked at White Castle and the sexual activities that occurred there.

We were laughing silently when Arlan looked at me and whispered, "I have to get my own room!"

Perhaps the hardest parts of that first hospital stay was being on the side away from the window and having no natural light. As the days wore on, we began drawing back the separating curtain more and more to get a glimpse outside.

Meanwhile, Alex was at my house with the kids, navigating homework, softball/baseball practice and various other activities. At least once each day, Rebecca would visit the hospital, frequently bringing food, and sit with Arlan while I ran home, took a shower, grabbed some hugs and kisses, and assured the kids that "Daddy was doing great!"

Devon came by so I could go into work for a few hours. When Rebecca brought the kids to the hospital, Arlan chose to visit with them in a family lounge rather than the room.

On his second day of chemo, I met them downstairs.

"How's Daddy?" Emma asked quietly.

"He's great," I said smiling, reassuringly.

Jonah hugged me hard and stuck very close to me as we silently rode the elevator up to the waiting room. Arlan sat there in his plaid pajama bottoms and a t-shirt that read "Screw Bone Cancer." He had ordered the shirt immediately from the web upon diagnosis and he dubbed it his cancer fighting shirt. He looked very much as he did on any weekend morning, with the exception of the IV and pole. He held out his arms and both Emma and Jonah collapsed into him taking up the rest of the small loveseat. I looked at my sister, who had turned away with tears in her eyes, as he began to quiz them on the happenings in their lives since he had last seen them.

That first hospital stay seemed endless. The dearth of light, the roommate, the lack of space and Arlan's increasing cabin fever all made me feel progressively more exhausted and stressed out. Added to my exhaustion was the lack of any place to sleep at the hospital.

I had promised Arlan to be with him every step of the way and stayed at the hospital the whole time. The first night I slept in the side chair with my feet propped on the corner of the bed. I woke up achy and had trouble standing straight. The second night, Arlan shifted over and silently lifted the covers. I climbed in next to him, trying to use as little of the bed as I could. I was overwhelmed with my constant worry for Arlan, my desperation to re-assure the kids, my fear about bringing him back to our less than pristine home, and my self-imposed need to continue working each day. As a result, I felt crippled by stress and anxiety, and numb, as if all I had to do was go through the motions each day. It wasn't that I was pretending to be okay, I really was okay. In my heart, I knew that as long as I insisted all was well, it would be. I simply could not allow myself to believe otherwise. When Arlan woke up nauseous on his first morning in the hospital and was dosed with anti-nausea meds, I took it in stride, feeling almost as if I were observing both him and myself from the outside.

On his third day of chemo, my mother and her husband got back from their cruise. Naturally, we were the first call she made as soon as they had cell service again. I explained what we had learned about the staging, emphasizing once again that this was going to be a tough fight but our confidence that he would win. My mom sent her love and assured me that they would catch a plane home quickly and be in Columbus by the next evening.

Late the following evening, my cell rang—my mother and step-father had arrived at the hospital. I gave them directions and met them on the way. I heard the ding of the elevator and looked across the walkway that bridged from the hospitals to the parking garage. As my mother rushed toward me, I again began to sob. Shaking off the tears more quickly this time, I led them up to Arlan's room explaining that he was experiencing some side effects and was sleeping deeply. Between the chemo and the anti-nausea medication he was out a good deal of the time. We silently entered the room and my mother, who had never been particularly close to Arlan, reached over and tenderly smoothed his brow. I took some rapid swallows to remain under control and led them to a small conference room nearby to show them the copies of x-rays, scans and other information I had amassed.

We also talked about what would happen after the five days of chemo were finished. My mother is a fastidious housekeeper to say the very least. Few things make her happier or prouder than sharing how, despite minimal sleep, her home gleams and shines. In all honestly, you can walk into her house and eat off ANY surface; it's that clean. Hearing that we assembled a workforce to get things straightened and sanitized at our place was like the mother ship calling her home. After the initial visit at the hospital, she took her rightful spot as general of the cleaning army. Although I recognized this was stressful for all those living and working at the house, I admit to taking considerable comfort knowing that she would be inspecting the progress on the home front.

As the first round of chemo drew to a close, we were visited by numerous medical professionals. Knowing that we were heading out soon, our spirits were high and we laughed with everyone who entered. The oncologist on call came in and once again examined Arlan's leg, feeling around the tumor and asking questions. When he remarked that things felt a little less tight, we took that as proof positive the chemo was working. The doctor also told us they would be scheduling Arlan for a lung biopsy the coming week. Arlan immediately tensed up and I flashed on the image of him sobbing following the fine needle biopsy. It continued to haunt me. The doctor assured us that Arlan would be out for this procedure. It was the only way to confirm that the cancer in his lungs was osteosarcoma, not another type, as typing affects treatment.

Before Arlan was released, we received a number of directives from the medical staff. Michelle had already explained that he would have his blood drawn weekly to monitor him and measure when his immune system bottomed out. The low point of the cycle was referred to as the nadir. Once he hit that, his system would begin to rebound. However, chemo had a cumulative effect, and the more rounds, he had, the longer it might take to reach nadir and the harder it would get for his system to recover. When the discharge nurse explained that the Neulasta shot Arlan was scheduled for would help him to hit nadir sooner and boost the rebound, we were eager for him to have it.

When she left, Arlan's roommate commented that the shots cost $5,000 each. Fortunately, after a brief challenge from our insurance company which initially claimed that Neulasta was an experimental drug, we managed to get it covered. I wondered if these shots were actually liquid gold and shuddered thinking about patients who were not insured.

Driving home together that evening felt surreal. Lack of sleep and general stress, plus having spent so much time in the dark hospital room, left me again, feeling almost as if I was on the outside watching myself. I couldn't wait to get back to familiar surroundings, but had trouble picturing what to do when I got there.

Although I appreciated the hard work everyone had put in getting the house ready for Arlan's homecoming, I am not proud to admit to my reaction upon arrival. When I opened the door to make sure the dogs were outside and Arlan could settle comfortably, the first thing I saw was the new welcome matt that someone had placed inside. I immediately picked it up and tossed it over my shoulder into the garage. While I understood the desire to provide something for people to wipe their feet on and avoid tracking stuff into the house, I was far more concerned about the stability of crutches on the matt and instantly deemed it unworthy of the risk. Although my actions were surely callous and hurtful to whoever had been thoughtful enough to place the matt, the act of tossing it over my shoulder provided a physical relief of all the stress I had accumulated in the hospital. Arlan came in and went immediately to the couch and both Emma and Jonah plopped down right next to him. My heart leaped in my chest, and I was overwhelmed with joy and gratitude that the first round was behind us, the chemo was working and we were all back under the same roof.

The next day we returned briefly to the hospital for the $5,000 shot, and Alex headed home for two weeks. Those first few nights at home the kids stuck very close to us, seeking constant hugs and attention. Arlan appeared only too happy to provide them. I was distracted, however, and shorter with my children than I wish now, in retrospect, I had been.

8

Life Continues, with Side Effects!

Everyone flourished with us back at home. Neither the dogs, nor the kids could get enough time or attention. Milo, our 3-year-old Yorkie Poo, was a mommy's boy all around, and now even more so, rarely leaving my lap if I was home and seated right next to me the rest of the time. Molly, our 3-year-old Great Dane, was Arlan's dog for sure.

She had come to us about a year and half earlier after our 13-year-old Siberian husky passed away. Nikita was Arlan's from before we met and he missed her terribly. When we began to talk about rescuing or adopting another large dog, Arlan did careful research online. He concluded that a Great Dane might be perfect for our family, but was concerned about how 12-pound Milo might react to having a "sibling" more than ten times his size. I read an ad on Craigslist that someone had a female Dane in need of a new home, and I called Arlan excitedly from work.

"I'm not sure we're ready," he said.

"At least go take a look," I pleaded. "We could take a ride out there this weekend."

"Oh no! No way are you going! You'll bring the dog home for sure, no matter what."

Realizing that he was likely correct and that my staying home was the only way to get him to go look at her, I agreed to attend Emma's softball game with Jonah that evening while Arlan and Milo took a ride over to see the dog. He only wanted to take Milo along to see how he'd manage with such a large dog and stressed to me several times that he was NOT bringing this dog home. He was simply checking it out as part of his research into the breed and made me promise not to tell the kids what he was doing.

About half way through Emma's game my cell phone rang—it was Arlan. "I have to bring this dog home."

"What happened?" I asked excitedly.

He sounded grim as he explained that the dog was in deplorable conditions, tethered to a tree with a metal chain looped around her neck. There was a dish in sight, but no water in it. She was filthy, had cuts and scratches all over, and you could count every rib. There was a kennel for her with no bottom tray just the metal webbing. The woman at the house claimed she was up to date on shots, but the vet records has been misplaced and she "could not recall" the name of the vet.

"I can't leave her like this, I just can't," he sighed.

So he loaded the dog into the car and headed home.

He called me again ten minutes later. By then the kids and I were home, and they were getting showered. "I bet she's dehydrated," Arlan said. "I'm going to pull over and give her just a little water. If she does okay with it, I'll give her more when we get home."

"What's her name?" I asked.

"The woman at the house called her Roxanne, but she doesn't respond to it. I like Molly, I've been calling her Molly."

"That's a sweet name."

"She's really dirty. We are going to have to keep her kenneled until she can get a bath," he announced. "We need to figure out the bottom of the kennel we can't let her sleep on the grate from the cage."

I agreed, put the kids to bed and then got out a thick rug from the kitchen and an old king sized comforter. When the garage door went up, I ran downstairs with it to greet our new potential family member. Milo came in first, looking fairly disgusted that his daddy was doting on this small horse. Then Arlan led Molly inside. She looked exactly as he described her.

"I don't think we should let her on the furniture," he said. "She's just so big, it seems like a bad idea."

"I think it may be a little late."

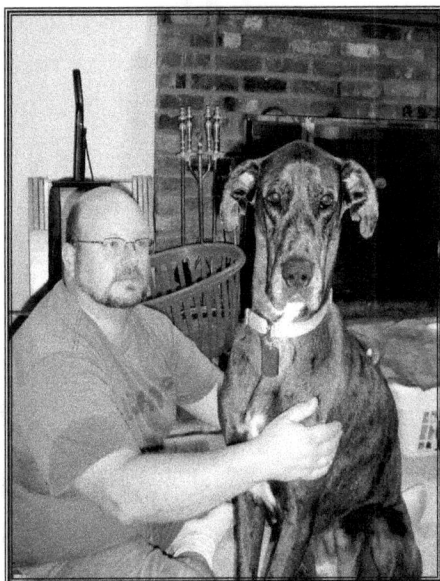

Molly had walked in, backed up to the couch and sat back much as a person would. We stood there looking at her, and she looked back at us with sad eyes. In that moment, I knew that she was home for good.

As Molly regained her health, she claimed her spot as the most loving and sweet member of our household, and she always looked at Arlan with the devotion of hero worship. He likely saved her life that night; she knew it and adored him.

On the advice of the oncologist, Arlan had been placed on temporary disability from work so he could concentrate all his energy on getting well. As he recovered from the chemo, he napped frequently. I often came home from work to find him and Molly stretched out together on the couch.

Arlan experienced many of the expected chemo side effects, but I remained matter of fact about the symptoms, observing with a weird sense of detachment. I also became fairly rigid about insisting on trying all the remedies I could discover. When he complained of nausea I got a cool washcloth and encouraged him to have a saltine, when he asked for words to be repeated or what the dialogue was on television, I silently turned up the volume. I morphed into a walking encyclopedia of chemotherapy side effect remedies. For me it felt as if our life was spiraling out of my control, but by equipping myself with knowledge I could hold back the tide.

By the beginning of the second week following chemo, Arlan really perked up. His hair continued to fall out at an impressive rate. We laughed and cringed as he lost some of his eyelashes, the hair on his toes and everything in between. Arlan joked that we needed a trip to the beach because his back would soon be hairless, referring to a time eleven years earlier when we took a trip to Myrtle Beach with some friends. The week before Arlan shared that he was self-conscious about the hair on his back and asked if I had ever used hair wax. I had not, but offered to get some so we could give it a try.

I bought the wax kit and we carefully read the instructions. I tried some on my calf while Arlan experimented with a small patch on his arm, and we agreed it wasn't too uncomfortable. He lay down on some towels on the family room floor. I heated the wax, straddled his legs and coated both sides of his back thoroughly with the warm substance. Then I laid the linen strips on top and rubbed them for maximum adhesion to the hair. After waiting the allotted time I held his skin firmly taught and pulled quickly on the first strip. Arlan screamed and bucked so hard that I was thrown off his legs and landed on the floor next to him.

"Holy crap that hurts!" he yelled.

"Oh my god, I'm so sorry," I gasped.

As Arlan slowly lowered himself back to the towels, the linen strip half dangling off his back, I noticed with dismay that he was bleeding where the wax had come off. After much urging and cajoling on his part, I finally agreed to finish the job. As Arlan braced himself, I pulled as gently as possible, tearing the remaining linen away and then wept quietly. Arlan immediately sat up and put his arms around me.

"Don't cry, baby," he said soothingly.

As I continued to weep, he collapsed in nearly hysterical laughter, observing between gasps that he was the one with the bleeding back and that I was the one who was crying.

9

Second Verse Same as the First

The following Monday we returned to the hospital for Arlan's lung biopsy. The coordinator from Dr. Neki's office expressed regret that he had to go through the procedure since the results were a foregone conclusion—it was nearly 100% certain that the cancer in his lungs was osteosarcoma—but it was a necessary formality to make sure everything was properly classified for insurance. In what felt like the blink of an eye, but was really two days later, we were back at the oncologist office to hear the results. As anticipated, it was osteosarcoma. I learned that when microscopic pieces of a cancer break off and metastasize to other parts of the body, it is actually the same as the original cancer. In Arlan's case, the bone tumor had traveled to his lungs and began to grow what was essentially cancerous bone there. I was both horrified and fascinated by this novel information.

The next round of chemo started a pattern that would soon become all-too-familiar—in and out of the hospital for a week or so each time, with the attendant frustrations of having to deal with the challenges of his port, the uncompromising admissions routines and a host of troubling side effects. We did warm to Dr. Neki who listened attentively before each admission as we catalogued the many side effects Arlan experienced, and constantly evaluated the cost versus benefits of the chemo. One time, he reminded us that hearing loss was most likely permanent and that we should keep him informed if it became extreme. When Arlan mentioned a swelling in his right foot, Dr. Neki ordered an ultrasound and discovered that he had developed a large clot behind his right knee and smaller ones in his left ankle.

The power port continued to be a challenge, but most pronouncedly during the second round. After various admission delays, we finally settled in a room and the nurse began the port access. As she laid Arlan flat on the bed and began to probe around the port on his chest, I saw him wince. She explained that she was feeling for the bumps that would guide her to the correct place to insert the needles, but that was no comfort. She was hurting him, and he had been hurt so much already. I felt a surge of protectiveness and told her that while we understood why she was doing it, she was still hurting him. She responded that enough time had passed from the port placement for Arlan to have healed. This did little to calm my anger at her lack of compassion.

After considerable prodding, she poked the needle into Arlan's chest and missed. She withdrew it and attempted to insert a new one into the other side. Again she missed. As she withdrew that one, both she and Arlan stiffened. I jumped to my feet and asked if perhaps there were someone else who could try as Arlan reached for my hand. The nurse explained that this was a super power port rather than the regular power port she was used to, which made it a bit more challenging. Moving between her and the bed I repeated my question.

Before we knew it, the on-call nurse for port issues, who identified herself as Mandy, came. She began to feel gently around Arlan's port and noted him wincing. Smiling kindly she suggested that we get some EMLA cream. Apparently, some people never stop experiencing sensitivity at the site of the port placement. If this prescription cream were applied about half an hour before the port was accessed, it should numb it enough to offer some relief. Suiting up into her sterile garb, she laid Arlan flat again, raised the bed and managed to access the port on both sides.

Following every two rounds of chemo, Arlan had another MRI and CAT scan to look at the tumor. Although they did not show any significant changes in his lungs or his leg, we were told that something positive seemed to be happening. Unfortunately, it was never enough to make a change, so we just kept going. During some rounds Arlan was so exhausted that he would nap in a recliner while we waited to be assigned a room.

I learned many lessons doing those long weeks in and out of chemo: EMLA cream should be applied no more than an hour before the port was accessed. Regardless of the skill of the assigned nurse, Arlan felt most comfortable when Mandy accessed his port, which helped him relax and made the process more successful. And we could call admissions on the mornings he was scheduled to start chemo, get his name on the list early, and have them notify us when they had a private room ready and he could check in.

Somehow we fell into a hospital routine. Nurses, patient assistants and doctors became familiar to us. We looked forward to seeing Michelle, our physician assistant, who bustled in daily, collapsed into a chair after examining Arlan and visited like a dear family friend. The rhythm of poking, prodding and taking of vital signs was no longer alien, and we settled comfortably into a private room.

Being in the family waiting rooms at a cancer hospital is much like joining a bizarre kind of fraternity or sorority. Sitting there, making phone calls, waiting for the restroom or just taking a few minutes alone to breathe, you hear the tearful calls others are making, observe the pale, shell-shocked faces of family members keeping vigil or reeling from recent bad news, and share the celebration of positive test results. Somehow, the barriers between strangers—color, religion, social and economic status—break down; health becomes paramount. As part of this group of scared and courageous people I learned where to get extra socks when we needed them; which floors had unlocked pantries stocked with popsicles and soda to settle upset stomachs; and where to find the only real privacy at the hospital—the family restroom on the first floor, which was all but abandoned at night.

The biggest nugget of wisdom I got was that rather than ordering meals from the kind dieticians who visited daily to try to find menu items Arlan could stomach, we could get meal tickets instead. The vouchers could be used in the hospital cafeteria and allowed him a wider variety of choices. Every morning after his vitals were taken and meds were dispensed at 6 a.m., I would trek downstairs and through the two other hospitals which attached ours to the cafeteria. There I would redeem our vouchers for a vanilla cream doughnut for Arlan and coffee and a bagel for me.

It was essential to get there on time or they would run out of his doughnut of choice, and I would not be able to get him to eat anything for hours. Also, I had to get back upstairs before someone showed up with a breakfast tray and removed the lid. The odors wafting into the room would make Arlan violently ill.

By the time we reached the fourth round of chemo, Arlan was eating virtually nothing. Very little tasted good to him; even the idea of food held limited appeal. I was constantly on the road, or asking someone else to drive to this place or that, chasing down some food he thought he might like to try. More often than not, he'd take only a bite or two and declare it tasted funny and be done.

The best time to get Arlan to eat well was when he was distracted by visitors during meals. Between chatting and engaging in the lives of others, he would eat much more. I often suspected this was out of habit more than hunger. As we sat at the table, he would eat without really thinking about it. Unfortunately, someone would invariably point out what a great appetite Arlan had and, for some reason, I often felt defensive; as if his having eaten well at this meal negated all the worrying and driving and attempting to tempt him with other food. In retrospect, I wish I had just enjoyed the moments when he was doing well and accepted them for what they were.

Meanwhile, I had become an expert at getting us settled into and out of hospital rooms. I had a bag packed with the pictures I used to decorate his hospital room, a few little candies to keep his throat wet, which he tolerated, and some magazines and other items we used at the hospital. I also kept parking passes, spare change, and a change of clothes for each of us in it. When the last bag of chemo was empty, I would retrieve an empty wheelchair and then sweep around the room in a clockwise direction, starting near Arlan's head, unplug chargers, gather pictures and other personal items which I loaded onto the wheelchair and pushed to the car. While Arlan waited to have his port de-accessed and his release paperwork processed, I'd move the car to a handicap spot close to the door and return to the room with the now empty wheelchair. After the first admission we never waited for an orderly to take us out. By the time the nurse came in with release papers, Arlan was in the chair, dressed and ready to go.

As we pulled away from the hospital, he would relax, and by the time we pulled into our own driveway 20 minutes later, he was a different man. His eyes would dance as he opened the door and put his arms around the kids. Then he would melt into the couch with our Great Dane cuddled by his side.

Late one afternoon while Arlan was napping at home, Scott called from Japan. He and Beth were thinking of coming to visit with their girls, Lauren and Lani, over the summer. Beth graciously offered to take my kids and all their cousins to Disney World for a week. I knew Emma and Jonah would be thrilled—they adore their cousins, Aunt Beth and of course Disney. Scott's plan was to meet up with his family in Ohio, spend a few days with Arlan, and then head to Pennsylvania to help his mom and sister; but he might just go to Pennsylvania directly as Arlan had seemed so positive when they spoke. I felt a prickle along my spine and asked just what Arlan had shared with him. Scott said that he knew Arlan had nodes in his lungs, but he was responding to the chemo and figured he would be having bone salvage surgery on his leg by the end of the summer. When I asked what he had been told about the prognosis, Scott repeated the party line we had been using.

In a rare moment of clarity, I swallowed hard and said, "I hate that I am telling you this, but that is not exactly what we are being told. The doctor's don't think Arlan will beat this, although we continue to believe that he will live for a good long time. At this point we are fighting for time…ideally many, many years. We know that this is a tough battle and he is fighting with everything he's got."

There were several seconds of silence and then I heard Scott's tearful voice. He had not quite understood the serious nature of the situation and would definitely be coming in. I could hear Beth softly crying on the line, too.

By then Arlan had awakened, and I turned the phone over to him. As I went to fold laundry, I felt sick to my stomach at the news I had just delivered. I wondered if Arlan had been less than honest with his mother, too; and even with himself. I'm not sure I did any better. At the time, I was unable to even consider what soothing lies I might be telling myself.

10

Getting Some Help

One Wednesday evening during a chemo session, I left Arlan at the hospital with a good friend of his and took Emma and Jonah to a support group for children of parents with cancer. While they worked on a craft project and spoke with the kids in their group, I sat in a circle with other adults: a mom who was fighting cancer, a mom who had recently beaten it, a care giver who was welcoming a young boy into her family because his mother (her best friend) was in the final stages of lung cancer, and a couple in which the husband and father was a survivor. The group was led by two social workers.

As we went around the circle to do introductions, I grew immediately hostile. I had brought my kids to get some help dealing with Arlan's illness but didn't want to delve into my own feelings. I found myself getting increasingly annoyed and uncomfortable despite maintaining my smile. I was jealous of those who had beat cancer and resentful that they were in the circle even as I offered congratulatory applause. The woman who was battling cancer was in bad shape and had a truly awful story, but I was too pre-occupied with concern about my kids to focus on what she was saying and found I lacked the emotional reserves to try.

When the woman with the dying friend started to speak, she quickly lost her composure and started to sob, and I got up and stepped into the ladies room. By the time I returned, she was weeping quietly. Then it was my turn. I provided an overview of my situation with calm detachment. The group leader asked me how I was feeling and I smiled and said I was concerned about how the kids were coping, but I was doing fine. She paused, apparently waiting for me to say something more, and when I did not, moved on. An hour and half dragged by as I attempted to look at without actually seeing the various group members.

Eventually we were joined by a young woman who identified herself as the leader of the kids group. She, another social worker and a handful of volunteers worked with the kids on crafts projects while talking about their experiences, fears and feelings.

Imagine my shock when she turned to me and said, "You must be Emma and Jonah's mom. They had a lot to say."

Apparently, my kids were feeling confused and nervous and didn't know how to start conversations with Arlan and me. While they heard us say that all was well, they felt frightened by how much time we were at the hospital and how quickly Arlan became sick after the first round of chemo. I listened quietly and asked her what I should do for them.

"Sounds like Arlan's pretty sick," she said gently.

"He is, but he'll get through it, it'll turn out fine."

She exchanged quick glances with the other social workers, then suggested I consider seeking family and maybe even individual counseling for the kids as well. "The more talking you all do the better for everyone," she assured me.

As we gathered our things, it occurred to me that my children would probably not want to come back to this gathering, and I was fine with that. Jonah generally avoided every social situation and Emma, despite being gregarious and extroverted, was never one to enjoy focusing on negative conversation.

The kids were quiet as we headed back to the car.

"How was that?" I asked.

"Really good," Emma responded.

"Really?"

"Yeah, I want to go every week."

"Okay," I responded evenly and turned to Jonah. "How about you?"

"Good," he said.

"Do you want to keep going?" I asked, sure he would either say no or at the very most give a non-committal shrug.

"Yes," he replied immediately.

I sat silently for a few minutes, stunned by their reactions. Finally I asked, "Want to talk about anything? Want to tell me about it?"

Neither of them did, and we rode the rest of the way home in silence.

I scheduled an appointment to see a family therapist the following week. I struggled considerably with what the best strategy for this counseling might be. Jonah is quite difficult to talk to, and it is always tough to predict how he will respond to someone he doesn't know. Also, I had my own questions regarding just what the counseling would accomplish. More than anything I wanted to offer the kids some sense of reassurance, but worried that the counselor would ask us to confront Arlan's mortality rather than help us be hopeful. I decided to go alone to the first appointment and bring Andy, the therapist, up to date on what we were facing.

"So what is it that you hope to get out of this counseling?" he asked.

With no hesitation, I explained that Arlan and I were certain that he would beat this, but that the kids were having to cope with significant changes in our home life in the meantime, and more were likely to come. Andy listened carefully. Then he looked up at me and calmly said that we may want to discuss what happens if Arlan doesn't make it. I shook my head resolutely. That was the kid's fear, but although things looked bad, we wanted them to believe that their daddy would get well.

"How does Arlan feel? How is he doing with all of this?"

"He has never been one to talk much about his feelings."

Andy suggested that it might be helpful to have Arlan join the conversation, and I assured him I would discuss it with him, although I doubted he would come. Andy offered to call Arlan and get his thoughts by phone, which seemed a reasonable compromise, and we scheduled for Emma and Jonah to come in the following week.

Naturally, when the appointment rolled around, I was in the midst of a rare productive day at work and left too late to pick up the kids at home and make it to Andy's office on time. I called Arlan and asked him to meet me with them. I was fully prepared to have him meet me in the parking lot, grab the kids and catch him up at dinner after the session. When I had mentioned his participating in the sessions, Arlan, as expected, had emphatically declined, but when I arrived in the parking lot to Andy's office, Arlan's van was empty. I found him and the kids in the waiting room. Without comment, I took a seat. When Andy called our last name, Arlan stood with the rest of us, and the four of us entered Andy's office together. Arlan and I each took one of the two couches in the room; Jonah sat close to me, and Emma parked herself with her dad.

The introductions were made, and to my shock Arlan turned to the kids and with no prompting began to talk. As I swallowed the lump in my throat, he said that he loved us beyond anything else and knew Emma and Jonah were likely confused and worried, but that he was ready to answer any questions they may have and hear whatever they might want to say. There was silence. Jonah looked at the picture hanging on the wall behind and over Arlan's head, but after a minute or so Emma began to speak.

Staring at her lap, she said, "Are you scared Daddy?"

"Scared of what?"

She shrugged and looked at him obliquely. The corners of her eyes welled up with tears.

Arlan focused on her intently before giving voice to what I suspect we were all thinking. "Am I scared of dying?"

Emma nodded as crocodile-sized tears ran down her cheeks.

Arlan never took his eyes off of her; he stretched his arm along the back of the couch and cupped her neck with his hand. In a gentle voice he said, "I'm not afraid to die, baby. As far as I know, no one is getting out of this world alive; everyone ever born, so far, has died, and I won't be any different. But I'm scared of leaving you and your brother. I'm scared of leaving your mom. I don't want you to grow up without me; I want to take care of all of you. I love you all so much, and it makes me scared and sad to think about you missing me. No matter what, I want you to know how much I will always love you and that I will always be with you."

I don't remember much more of what was said that day. I remember looking at Jonah and seeing the tears in his eyes and handing out tissues all around. I remember the way Arlan held me as I stood up to leave when our session had ended. And I remember feeling humbled by his ability to make a sacrifice for the kids' well-being. In all of the 17 years we had been together, talking about his feelings always represented the *last* thing he ever wanted to do; but for Emma and Jonah he did it with compassion and grace. What I did not understand then was that Arlan was changing. By then I think he already knew his days were numbered and he was preparing us for the inevitable.

This was perhaps the beginning of his hope transforming from beating his disease to leaving us in a healthy, loving space. It was the first of what in retrospect, I can see were many instances of Arlan attempting to move our family forward and prepare us for the end.

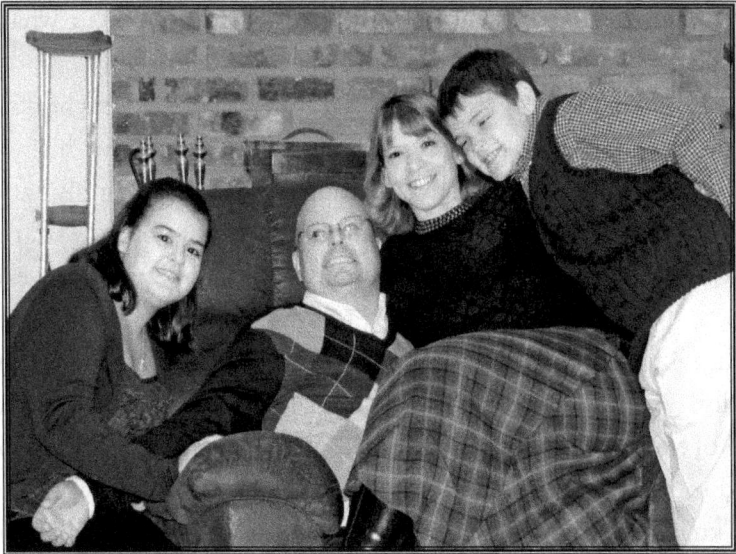

11

Clear as Mud

We continued to attend sessions with Andy as a family around Arlan's chemo. Although Arlan had all the usual side effects—nausea, trouble eating, trouble hearing, confusion, dizziness, bloody noses and fatigue—we took it all in stride. During one chemo cycle Arlan had required a blood transfusion as his platelets dropped to a dangerously low level, and we were not too surprised when he needed another between chemo weeks. It did, however, present something of a logistical problem.

I was in my office when my phone rang and Arlan cheerfully informed me that he had been scheduled for a transfusion and would be leaving soon for the hospital. He had to get there right away as he would be getting at least two bags of blood and they were holding a chair for him at the lab. I told him to sit tight and called a neighbor who was kind enough to run him over to the hospital (she got lost on the way home).

I left my office a short time later and found him sitting in the outpatient chemo lab hooked up to a bag of blood which was dripping into his arm. He opened his eyes when I came behind his curtain and held up his arm, explaining that they hadn't been able to get the port working. I patted his arm and realized, despite seeing him every day, just how much weight and muscle tone he had lost.

Later that evening I made a conscience effort to look at him and noticed that all his hair was gone. Perhaps for the first time I really saw how different he looked with his sallow, hairless skin.

Following four rounds of chemo, it was once again time for scans, and we were excited to finally be scheduled to see a thoracic surgical oncologist (the lung guy). As we sat in the waiting room of his office, my leg bobbed up and down and Arlan swallowed convulsively—physical manifestations of just how nervous we were. We both had computers open on our laps and stared at the screens without really seeing them. Neither of us ever moved our mouse.

Finally, we were escorted to an examining room where we went through our routine: Arlan made himself comfy on the table while I gathered our bags behind my chair. Then I slipped his gray hoodie off his shoulders and wrapped myself in it, breathing in his familiar scent and heat.

The doctor who came in, a man in his early to mid-40's, had a serious expression. He had reviewed all the scans and he didn't have much to offer. The doctor explained that given the amount of cancer in Arlan's lungs and leg, he was not a viable candidate for surgery at this time. Arlan looked fixedly at a point just outside the window as his eyes began to tear up.

Since we already knew that there were multiple nodes in Arlan's lungs, I began to ask pointed questions. We learned that there were more than 30 nodes; in a typical osteosarcoma case the number was three or four. The nodes ranged from a few millimeters in diameter to about the size of a quarter, and there were likely many more not yet visible to the naked eye. While it was theoretically possible to remove all of them and have enough lung left to sustain life, the problem for Arlan was that they were not in one specific section but spread throughout. If they were removed, there would be no one area of his lungs large enough to provide him with clean oxygen.

Arlan rallied and began to ask questions of his own. "How soon could we start trying to get the largest nodes out?"

"Not that simple" the doctor said.

In a typical surgery, he could remove four or five nodes at the most. To get all of Arlan's would take at least six major surgeries, without a guarantee that no additional nodes would grow or that there would be enough lung for him to live.

"Well I guess we better start soon," Arlan said.

"What about a lung transplant?" I asked.

The doctor shook his head sadly. The existence of all the nodes in Arlan's lungs was evidence that the cancer was traveling from his leg around his body. Until the "source" was addressed and stopped leaking cells, there was little point in trying to develop a plan for the lungs.

We left with heavy hearts and drove in silence to our next appointment with the original orthopedic oncologist, the first specialist we had seen. This time we didn't bother with computers and sat in the waiting room hand in hand. Arlan sweated as I sat shivering in his jacket.

The news from Dr. Mayerson was if anything even more confusing than what we had heard from the lung doctor. After reviewing the scans and examining Arlan's leg, he assured us that something was happening as a result of the chemo. He showed us a printout of the recent scan and where there was some necrosis (evidence of dead cancer cells)—in the tumor. Yet, the tumor was not shrinking and due to its positioning, there was not a "clear margin"—enough tissues around the tumor to cut it out completely—which would allow for a limb salvage procedure. Because the tumor had enveloped a major artery, there was no way to remove it all. Some would have to be left to preserve the artery, which of course meant an increased threat of new cancer growth.

With no hesitation whatsoever Arlan looked at the doctor and said, "Just take the damn leg."

He looked over at me and I nodded my head in agreement. I turned back to the doctor and assured him that we were prepared for Arlan to lose the leg; we just wanted him to be well.

Dr. Mayerson looked from Arlan to me and back at Arlan again. "This is a very complex issue," he said. "An amputation is major surgery; not just major surgery, giant, huge surgery. And ultimately it will not save your life." Smiling kindly, he continued, "There is just too much cancer in your lungs. Removing the leg at this point will not make a difference."

I wanted to scream, but I quietly asked how that could be since the thoracic surgeon just this morning had told us to come back once the source was addressed.

"Well that's the thing," Dr. Mayerson explained, tugging gently at his collar and running his hand through his hair repeatedly. "We really can't address the source because of the lungs."

12

Expanding the Team

Later that afternoon, I started to form a plan. If the folks at Arlan's cancer hospital couldn't find a way to cure him, then I would. I hit the Internet once again. This time instead of just reading sites for information, I began joining every group I could find that was associated with bone cancer or sarcomas. I posted the question everywhere I could think of: Where should an adult osteosarcoma patient go for options? As I went back and re-read articles I began taking note of the citations for authors, who had conducted trials and studies, and followed them to the national institute of health where I searched for current studies.

For days on end, I read until I could barely keep my eyes open. I made lists and pursued leads. I called several sarcoma centers around the country, and facilities in France and Japan as well, but nowhere in the world was there a clinical trial specific to Osteosarcoma for adults. This was terribly discouraging for me and devastating for Arlan. When he turned on the television or the radio, he'd see and hear about the globe painted pink for breast cancer awareness while he and millions of others fought rare and aggressive cancers in virtual invisibility and silence. Not that we didn't support the fight against breast cancer, but the total omission on rare cancer was frustrating. Arlan once shared with me that the pink shirts and ribbons had become offensive to him because it seemed that by supporting breast cancer all the others were ignored. To this day I remember that and try to be inclusive in the cancer fighting garb and symbols I wear.

Speaking to countless research centers, I ended every conversation by asking who else I should be speaking to. One name I heard over and over was Dr. Peter Anderson at the MD Anderson Cancer Center in Texas. His name was familiar to me from much of the research about Osteosarcomas it was regularly referenced in articles and studies. Although he worked with children, I was assured by several people that if I could get in touch with him, he likely would see Arlan. I began a campaign to make that happen, calling and emailing his office several times a day for about a week.

One day just as I was getting ready to leave my office for a meeting, my cell phone rang with an unknown number. A somewhat high voice asked for Rachel Silsdorf.

"This is she,"

"Hi, it's Dr. Pete," the caller said

"Who?" I asked, not registering that the man who had become a legend in my mind could be calling me personally.

"Dr. Pete, Dr. Anderson, from MD Anderson in Houston," he said uncertainly. "I believe you have been leaving me messages."

"Oh yes," I replied as my knees gave out and I sank back into my seat. In an instant, everything I wanted to discuss was gone from my head as if it had never existed.

Dr. Anderson must have this experience a lot because he took up the conversation effortlessly and asked questions about what had been done so far, exactly who we were seeing and what we knew.

"How soon can you get here?" he asked.

I felt my eyes tear up as I tried to respond.

Arlan was scheduled to start his next round of chemo the following week, and Dr. Anderson felt that should continue. His coordinator,

Gina, would get in touch with me to get Arlan scheduled for a visit at the clinic as soon as he finished the next round. Dr. Anderson agreed that amputating the leg was imperative and offered to set us up with a surgeon in Texas. We also discussed some experimental chemo regimens after Dr. Anderson pointed out that Arlan was approaching the lifetime maximum dose of the most effective known for Osteosarcomas. Before hanging up, he, kindly but gently explained that for a typical Osteosarcoma patient with lung metastases, the five-year life expectancy was about 10 to 12 percent, and that given the number of nodes in Arlan's lungs, anything he did would be to help him get into that group.

As promised, Gina contacted me several hours later. She not only efficiently provided lists of everything I would need to do and send to make the visit happen, she also provided practical ideas to help Arlan in the meantime. She suggested trying frozen drinks, smoothies, shakes, ices—the colder they were the better they'd feel on the throat and the easier they'd go down –whatever I could get him to drink. Plastic utensils would combat the metallic taste of food. A pillow between the box spring and the mattress under his head would help with some of the nausea and heartburn. Great suggestions! I used them all.

For the first time in my life without even considering the cost, I called an airline and booked tickets to Houston. One of our best friends was originally from there, and her mother, Mary, who my kids call Grandma, still lived there. We made arrangements for her to pick us up at the airport. Although she wanted us to stay with her, I thought it would be easier to be at a hotel near the hospital. Arlan became exhausted so quickly by then, and since he would be just off chemo, I would be pushing him in a wheelchair most of the trip.

I arranged for wheelchairs by contacting the airline and each of the airports we would visit. I learned that this could not be done via the Internet, so I called and waited through countless automated voice systems. When I finally reached a live person, I carefully wrote down the name and date. I had begun to carry a notebook with all of Arlan's medical records, and I added a spiral notebook to record all the details of the many calls I made each day.

Although Dr. Anderson had been clear that he did not believe he would be able to save Arlan's life, my conversation with him was rejuvenating. I felt hopeful and excited again as I began to research the drugs he had mentioned, sent records, followed up on his recommendations and got ready for our visit to Houston.

13

Adventures in Chemo

The following Tuesday, as usual, we checked in with the oncologist before going to our next round of chemo. Despite our original impression of him as overly negative, Dr. Neki had grown on us. His gentle, quiet, yet firm demeanor had been off-putting until we came to understand it was born of patience and compassion. Of all the doctors we saw, only Dr. Neki looked us in the eye and acknowledged our anger and frustration. We counted on him to tell us the hard truths; we believed he was absolutely on our side. When we described our visits with the two surgeons, he explained that neither of his colleagues wanted to come right out and say it, but what they were really telling us was that surgery would be pointless.

"It's my only option," Arlan insisted.

"No, this is not an option," Dr. Neki responded emphatically. "The surgery will make you sicker, weaker and nothing will be gained. If you were my brother, I would say no."

Excitedly, I shared with him my conversation with Dr. Anderson and our plan to see him. Dr. Neki's enthusiasm matched our own as he asked many questions and began taking notes.

"I will call and e-mail him," he promised. "We will work with him any way we can so you can be close to home and your kids".

Then he began his regular examination and questioning of Arlan about the state of his health during the last two weeks. Arlan and I shared that we had noticed a marked decline in his hearing. He routinely asked for people to repeat themselves, was unable to hear the phone ringing, and listened to the TV at high volumes. Dr. Neki smiled sadly. After the physical exam he said that we needed to change the chemo regimen. The hearing impairment was a permanent side effect and Arlan would not recover what he had lost. Continuing the current meds could result in a complete hearing loss. It would be better to switch to a new drug which had shown some promise with sarcoma patients. This was the same drug that Dr. Anderson had mentioned to me, so I was anxious for Arlan to try it.

We checked in for that round of chemo with rejuvenated hope for the first time in quite a while. We were excited about being assigned the largest single room in the unit. It was spacious and I had a cot instead of the usual, uncomfortable chair. I actually slept well that first night secure in the knowledge that we would leave for Houston the following week and that Arlan was receiving the drug that Dr. Anderson had recommended.

When I woke on the second morning, Arlan was still sleeping. Although the nurse came in to check his vitals and dispense some meds, he did not really wake up much. I wasn't alarmed—he had become increasingly fatigued as the weeks had passed and I approached the bed myself to try to wake him. He did raise his head and turned toward me, but when his eyes opened, he looked at me with anger.

"What?" he groused as I tried to get him to sit up to take meds and started to raise the head of his bed. "Stop!"

"Take it easy babe," I said reassuringly.

Focusing on my face, he began to relax. "Sorry," he told me.

When I returned from my morning trip to the cafeteria, Arlan did not want to eat his doughnut or sip his juice. I finally cajoled him into taking two bites of a bagel before he went back to sleep. In the early afternoon he woke up and went into the bathroom, where he stayed for well over an hour. I knocked on the door intermittently, asking if he was okay. After the third time, the patient assistant knocked to check on him.

When Arlan finally came out and we repeatedly asked if everything was okay, he looked at us oddly and said, "Why wouldn't it be?"

Then he returned to bed and went to sleep.

The next morning, my friend Lisa came by the hospital to sit with Arlan for the day so I could go to work. I rushed into the parking garage and called Arlan's Mom from the car. I told her how worried I was about him not eating or drinking the last few days.

"Get him a strawberry banana smoothie," she advised.

One of the things I love most about my mother-in-law is that she is a perpetually sunny person. Despite catching more than her share of bad luck from the universe, she chooses joy and reflects a bright disposition most of the time.

But as I drove out of the garage that day, I said to her, "Something's not right."

"Strawberry banana smoothie," she advised again.

I stayed at work for several hours, but could not shake the ominous feeling. As I headed back toward the hospital, I made a quick detour to pick up a strawberry banana smoothie. When I returned to Arlan's room, I found things much as I had left them. Lisa told me that he had woken once or twice, but said little or nothing despite her attempts to engage him. He hadn't eaten or drunk anything and hadn't acknowledged the staff much when they came in.

When I went to the bed to wake Arlan, he opened his eyes and snarled, "I'm awake and I can hear you."

"Great," I said. "Your Mom wants you to drink this."

Arlan looked at the smoothie I placed on the tray table as if I were attempting to feed him battery acid and turned his head away from us.

Ignoring him, Lisa and I began to chat quietly until Arlan's IV pole began to beep. Having spent considerable time in the hospital over the past few months, we were used to the intermittent beeping when an air bubble formed, a bag was low on liquid, or there was a non-specific malfunction. Arlan reached over, pushed the call button and when he got a response from the intercom he said his IV was beeping.

"We'll send your nurse in," the voice over the intercom promised.

Approximately 15 seconds later, Arlan pushed the call button a second time. When the voice again responded, he held the remote up to the beeping IV pole and roared, "THIS IS WHAT I AM LISTENING TO!"

Lisa and I stared at each other in horrified silence as a nurse rushed in and silenced the beeping. I stood up to walk her outside as we both shook our heads in shock over behavior that so was so foreign to Arlan it made him almost unrecognizable. When I returned to the hospital room, he had again retreated to the bathroom. This time it took over two hours to coax him out.

That night, I found myself once again unable to sleep. Arlan had bought me a Kindle for Mother's Day and I lay in my cot, reading through the night, listening to Arlan's breathing machine. Around three a.m. his IV pole began to beep again. I lay there for a minute waiting for him to hit the silencer and call for the nurse, but he did neither.

"Hit the button babe," I said.

"I can't," he responded. "Hit the nurse call button" I coaxed again.

"No, I can't. They're out there."

"Who?" I asked, getting up and heading to the bed to silence the beep myself.

As I got close to the bed, Arlan grabbed my wrist. "No!" he told me. "Stop it!"

I tried to pull my wrist away, but he wrenched it, pulling me close with much more force than I thought him capable of, given his lack of food for three days. He had never been one to act out violently.

"Arlan, you're hurting my arm."

From the corner of my eye I saw his other arm move toward me. I ducked down next to the bed to avoid the blow and managed to pull my wrist free. Then I crawled toward the door to get help. When I returned with a nurse, Arlan was once again asleep, and she reset the pole. The next morning when Arlan awoke briefly, he had no memory of the scuffle. Despite the black and blue marks on my wrist, I chalked it up to his being not really awake and acting out a nightmare.

Again Arlan slept most of the day. When the nurse practitioner and doctors came for rounds, he lay listlessly on the bed throughout the exam. Afterwards I stepped into the hall and spoke to Chad, the nurse practitioner. My skin felt itchy and I had a convulsive need to swallow as I implored him to help me understand why Arlan had become so unresponsive. He explained once again that chemo has a cumulative effect—something I had been hearing often—and suggested gently that at some point I might want to consider palliative care. I shuddered at the thought of no longer actively fighting the disease. It felt disloyal even having this discussion and I quickly ended it. I headed back into Arlan's room and sat silently on my cot in the dark room for several hours.

That was the final day of the new chemo, which required yet another new drug and an additional two-day hospital stay to flush it all from his system and protect his kidneys. Initially, I was concerned because we were scheduled to leave for Texas early the following week, but given how sick Arlan had been during this round, I felt relieved to have more time with other people around. As that day wore on, Arlan became a little more himself. He spoke to me more and was kinder. He also tried a few sips of the drinks I brought him, but spent another extremely lengthy period in the bathroom. Finally that night, he drifted into what appeared to be a more restful sleep with no murmuring or tossing.

When he woke up the next morning he ate some of his doughnut and sipped some juice. The doctors came in on their rounds, and I shared with them that Arlan seemed more himself. Arlan agreed that he was feeling pretty good as one of the doctors turned to me and asked if he had been hallucinating.

I responded sarcastically, "Contrary to popular opinion, I am not actually inside his head. I don't know." But I did relay the "nightmare."

Shortly after the doctors left, Arlan said, "You know, I think maybe I have been hallucinating."

"Oh, why is that?"

"Well, every time I go in the bathroom, I have the sense there is someone there to greet me. I kept wondering why you were making such a big deal about me spending so much time in there, because it wasn't like I was alone. Now that I think about it, though, I don't think there really was ever anyone else there."

I was so stunned I sat there in silence for several seconds. Then I jumped up, and ran out into the hall to the find the doctor. I dragged him back into the room and had Arlan repeat what he'd just told me. This time with more conviction, Arlan re-iterated that it was unlikely that there was an actual person in the bathroom with him. I began to shiver and quickly donned an extra layer of clothes. Following this revelation, Arlan was whisked downstairs for an MRI of his brain. Chad assured me that in all likelihood there was nothing to worry about. Osteosarcomas rarely, if ever, metastasized to the brain. Chances were that Arlan's behavior was a toxic reaction to the new meds, but they needed to look just to be sure. I sat in his hospital room and felt myself shaking in fear as I waited for Arlan to return and learn what they found. I couldn't imagine how much tougher this fight would be if his brain was infected and I was left with the stranger of the last several days. I called and left a message for Gina at Dr. Anderson's office, letting her know what had been going on and that I was worried about us making it to Texas. I stood up in anticipation as Arlan was brought back. The MRI showed nothing unusual. I felt myself sink into the chair in relief as Chad confirmed that all the weird behaviors were attributable to the new medication.

As the hours passed, Arlan seemed more and more himself. He began to tell jokes and engaged in conversation with each person who came in the room. Shortly after my sister arrived with our children and dinner, however, he became violently ill on the way to the bathroom. The suddenness shocked all of us. One second he seemed fine, and the next he and the floor were covered in vomit. No sooner had we cleaned up and he was back in bed than he began throwing up again. The nurse gave him a second shot of anti-nausea medication, which had the effect of almost instantly knocking him out.

Arlan slept fitfully through the night, but woke up seemingly refreshed. He was in surprisingly good spirits, and I felt like I had been given a reprieve. I was profoundly grateful to have him back and found myself constantly kissing him, talking incessantly, eager for the sound and comfort of his voice. But when he ate half of a dry bagel for breakfast, within 15 minutes he threw up once again.

When the doctor came in for rounds, he confirmed that the brain scans were clear. He was certain that the hallucinations and nausea were the result of toxicity issues with the new chemo meds.

I called Gina in Texas to ask what this news might mean for us moving forward. Together she and I made the decision to postpone the trip to Houston. Fortunately, Arlan was in a medication induced sleep as I sat by the window and silently cried while I waited on hold with the airline to change our flights.

By late the next morning Arlan managed to keep a few sips of ginger ale down with the assistance of oral anti-nausea meds. Michelle, our PA was back on shift by this point. My relief at seeing her was nearly physical. She was much more than just part of the medical team; she had become like family to us. When she walked in the room, I jumped up from my chair and hugged her. She perched on a chair listening carefully as we filled her in on the events of the past few days. In turn, she shared her adventures parenting her sons, which made us comfortable and feel closer to her.

The thing about Michelle was she didn't hold back. In kind, but clear terms she told us what we needed to know. "There are lots of ways we can adjust the doses," she said. "It will be up to Dr. Neki, but maybe this is not the drug for you. At this point, we just don't know."

I told her that we were anxious to get home to our children, and she agreed that it was time for Arlan to get out of the hospital.

She turned to him and said, "Okay, big guy, make you a deal. Try a few bites of toast, keep it down and you're free. I'll bust you outta here."

By the time the kids finished school that day we were home. Although we had only been in the hospital two extra days, it felt as if we had been away forever.

14

Air Bubble

I called Dr. Neki early the next morning. One of the things I loved about him was that he always called me back, not an assistant or a nurse. Although there were plenty of small questions or issues they addressed, when big problems arose or big decisions had to be made, he was accessible. Together we decided that we would postpone Arlan's next chemo for a week so that he would have a little extra recovery time after this episode before making the trip to Houston. Dr. Neki suggested we repeat his scans before we went so we would have recent ones done on the same machines.

With renewed hope and excitement we packed for our trip to Houston.

On the Friday before, I took Arlan over for his scans and then headed to the office for the afternoon. I came home and was surprised to find him lying on the bed with his eyes closed but clearly awake. I could see that he was agitated and touched my hand to his forehead.

"What's going on?"

"Neki called, I have a pneumothorax and he wants me to come back to the hospital."

"A what?"

"Some kind of an air bubble in my lungs. I told him no way, I'm going to Texas."

"Hang on. We need to know a little more about this before we decide."

"I knew you'd say something like that," Arlan accused and got up from the bed and walked across the room without his crutches.

"Arlan, get your crutches, come on, just give me a second here, let me figure out what this is, what this means," I pleaded.

"Dammit!" Arlan muttered, "I am not going back to that fucking hospital. Damn Neki just doesn't want me to go to Houston."

While he grabbed one of his crutches and began pacing around the room, repeating the accusation, I got out the laptop to look up pneumothorax.

Arlan said, "The thing is I can't fly. Neki said that changing air pressure is the problem. He wants me to come in so they can get a second look."

"So they don't want to keep you?"

"I don't know," he admitted, "but I am not going in at all, fuck it. I'm going to Texas anyway."

"Well, if the issue is that you can't fly, we'll drive." I quickly calculated that if we left that evening and even made frequent stops I could get him to Texas in time for Monday morning's appointment.

"You're too tired and you hate to drive" he responded.

"Doesn't matter," I said with growing confidence, "I can do it, if this is what it takes, I can get you there."

"Okay. Call Neki, tell him we are going to drive. Tell him I will come in for a minute so he can listen to my lungs on our way out of town."

As I picked up my phone to call the doctor, Arlan headed downstairs to call Alex and talk with the kids about our change in plans.

Unfortunately, when I reached Dr. Neki, I learned that the facts as Arlan had heard them were somewhat skewed. The scans had shown a large air bubble in his right lung, but the problem wasn't simply a matter of changing altitudes. The air bubble was quite large and filled with fluid. It is not uncommon for the bone growing in the lungs with metastatic Osteosarcomas to pierce the sac that surrounds the lungs and allow air to collect between the chest wall and the lungs. This situation could easily become deadly in a matter of minutes if the air pocket began to expand. Arlan needed to be admitted to the hospital right away.

When I tried to convince him that I could drive Arlan to Texas after dropping by his office, he said, "I strongly advise you to bring him into the hospital immediately. If it were my brother, he would already be here. I know you are disappointed, and he is scared and angry, but this can kill him, and very quickly."

From his tone and intensity, I finally understood and went downstairs to face Arlan.

I found him in the family room with the kids on the couch. They all stared at me, sensing that I had something so say.

"Arlan, I spoke to Dr. Neki." I began.

Before I could formulate exactly what to say, he dropped his head to his chest and sighed loudly. "We're not going to Texas."

I shook my head. My throat felt tight and I had to squeeze out the words to explain why not and that we should head to the hospital. Jonah got up and went to the basement. Emma looked at Arlan and cuddled into his side. Again he sighed loudly and held her against him. "Okay" he finally said.

Arlan was admitted into the hospital that afternoon. Once again, I called Gina to share our news. This time Dr. Anderson got on the phone himself. He agreed that there was no way for us to make the trip and suggested that Arlan's disease was progressing quickly.

"I wish I could have helped," he told me, "but you are welcome to keep sending test results and I will offer any input I can."

I begged him not to give up; we would reschedule the trip again as soon as Arlan was released.

However Dr. Anderson explained that now that he had developed one pneumothorax, he was at increased risk for additional ones. He urged me not to risk such a long and taxing trip considering that he didn't really think at this point he had much to offer anyway. We might want to think about some of the clinical trials for general sarcomas being done in Michigan to buy some time. I hung up feeling utterly defeated.

When I returned to Arlan's room trying to figure out how to tell him the bad news, I found him sitting up in bed with several nurses around him. He appeared to be enjoying the attention. As I came in, everyone got quiet. My face must have shown how upset I was because the room cleared quickly. I sat down at the end of the bed facing Arlan as I had so many times before and shared briefly what Dr. Anderson had said. His face fell into despair and he grew very quiet and did not respond.

A short while later a doctor came in and introduced herself as a lung specialist. She explained that they believed the fluid in the pneumothorax was likely cancerous. After some discussion with her group, however, they had come to the conclusion that there was no point in taking a sample and having it analyzed. The risk of puncturing the lung or the membrane leading to a collapsed lung was too great. Given how diseased Arlan's lungs were already, doing anything which could further damage them was simply not worth it. Her preferred course of action would be to push oxygen into his lungs by placing a tube in his nostrils. It would put pressure on the chest wall and force the air pocket to absorb. They would be taking another chest X-ray shortly and then carefully monitor the progress with additional chest X-rays. Because they were trying to force the lungs to inflate as much as possible, Arlan was placed on the highest flow of oxygen available. He also received an oxygen monitor on his finger. Should his blood oxygen level begin to fall, it would likely be the only indicator that he was in distress, at which point they would proceed with an emergency surgical intervention.

Arlan tolerated this monitoring fairly well, although he delighted in placing the oxygen monitor on my finger or Emma's saying he was tired of wearing it and we should "take it for a while". He particularly loved putting it on my finger and the alarm with which the nurses would run into the room when my blood oxygen was lower as I have always had asthma. This never failed to delight Arlan, who would cackle gleefully before they put the monitor back on his finger.

I admit I perked up a bit when I heard surgery, not because I wanted him to have to have it, but because my immediate thought was they could cut out some of the tumors in the process. It must have shown on my face because the doctor explained that we wanted to avoid surgery at all cost. Surgical options included placing a small tube to drain the air bubble, then tacking the lung to the chest wall; or draining the air bubble and then bonding the lung to the chest cavity by creating scar tissue that basically cements the lung in place. While the idea of preventing future occurrences was appealing, both surgeries sounded gruesome and painful, and neither included a reduction in the cancer.

Arlan seemed unfazed by any of this news and asked how soon he would be able to travel. Once the doctor left the room I again shared what Dr. Anderson had said. Arlan listened quietly, then turned away from me for several moments.

When he turned back he said, "I have to get to Texas, this guy is my only chance."

"Don't think like that" I begged.

"I have to, we have to be realistic, things are getting worse. We need a miracle. I need to buy time; as much as I can."

He pulled me toward him and I climbed into the bed next to him and held on tight. I can't say for sure who was comforting whom. Feeling his arms around me and the steady rise and fall of his chest was a balm to my soul. Looking back, I think that Arlan was buying time to offer comfort to me and to the kids. He had become so thoughtful and focused in his interactions with us and other family and friends, as if he were aware of exactly how much each interaction would replay in years to come. His hope for our happiness and well-being was becoming an almost tangible part of how we related to each other.

Over the next three days I became adept at reading Arlan's chest X-rays. Fortunately, the hospital had a mobile X-ray cart which would get wheeled in twice a day. From the safety of the hallway, I would watch the screen over the technicians' shoulders to visually measure the size of the air pocket. Slowly it began to absorb, and Arlan was again released from the hospital.

Now that visiting Texas seemed to be pretty much off the table, I was at a loss to envision a route to cure. When we returned to the oncology clinic to meet with Dr. Neki, he suggested that the tumors had likely shrunk as much as they ever would and that Arlan had now reached his lifetime maximum for the drug that is most effective in fighting Osteosarcoma. He again broached the subject of palliative care and even offered to give us the names of hospice agencies, but I politely and emphatically told him that we were not convinced that we had reached that stage. I looked at Arlan as I said it and saw him sit a little straighter. The tension seemed to drain from his shoulders as he gave me a small nod.

In response, Dr. Neki suggested an alternative regimen of chemo that could be administered on an outpatient basis. He smiled reassuringly at Arlan. While this was not as effective as what he had been getting, it was worth a try while he continued to look for alternatives. When I asked how he knew that the tumors would not get any smaller, he showed us the reports from the various scans side by side. I questioned why Arlan had only had one PET scan, and Dr. Neki explained that it is used simply to show if there is cancer present in the body, while the MRI and CAT scans are the real monitors.

Referring to my notes from an earlier conversation with Dr. Anderson, I pointed out that he had specifically mentioned the need to repeat the PET scan because it is the best measure of live cancer in the body when it comes to Osteosarcomas. Thumping his leg, Dr. Neki looked at Kay, his physician's assistant, smiled, said that Dr. Anderson was the leading expert and told her to order the test. He shook Arlan's hand and patted his shoulder as they headed out of the room. Arlan stood up and wrapped me in a hug, murmuring thank you's into my hair.

It turned out that Dr, Anderson was correct. When the PET scan came back, it showed less live cancer in the body than Dr. Neki had been expecting. Arlan was again admitted to the hospital with a new four day chemo regimen this time—not as aggressive as the original, but tougher than the outpatient would have been.

15

The Bone Gives Out

Arlan was pleased to be home in time for the "big game" the day after his release from the hospital when he finished with the new chemo. Following a tradition begun with my father and my sister's ex-husband, he considered every Ohio State University game a "big game" and watched them with enthusiasm. He woke in unusually fine spirits, the new regimen having been significantly less intense, and he reported that he was feeling good. Emma was out babysitting and Jonah was in the basement, playing with a friend. I made Arlan some snacks and decided to go out shopping at a nearby Target, to enjoy a few rare minutes by myself. As I began to browse mindlessly, relishing the solitude, I heard my cell phone ring in my purse. When I managed to fish it out, I saw that I missed a call from Arlan and immediately called back.

He answered right away. His voice sounded tense and high pitched.

"What's wrong? I asked, immediately on guard.

"I broke my leg."

He had been easing himself down into his recliner when he felt a sharp pain and his leg gave out from under him, sending him sprawling to the floor. He was still lying there.

"How do you know it is broken?

He simply responded, "It is."

I believed him. "Have you called 911?

"No, I didn't think of that; I called you."

I told him to stay where he was and call 911.

I was already running toward my car.

As I drove home, I phoned my sister and when she answered, I screamed, "Come quick, I need you to stay with the kids, come right now, oh shit, come quick," and hung up.

In my mind, the call went differently. I thought I said, "Arlan fell and thinks his leg is broken, I am on my way to the house to meet the ambulance. I need you to come stay with Jonah and Devlin.

Later, Rebecca told me what I had really yelled at her and how frightened she had been.

When I got home, I pulled up right behind the ambulance and jumped out of the car, leaving my purse and the car door open on the street. As I ran into the family room, I heard the EMTs asking Arlan questions. He was calm but pale, even for him, and his right thigh was quite swollen.

As one EMT began to gently probe his leg, I turned to the other and said "He has cancer in that leg. He was released from the James Hospital last night following chemo. He needs to go to OSU."

The man looked at me and calmly said, "Ma'am, there's a home game," as if no further explanation were required.

I repeated Arlan's status and the need for him to go to OSU. This time the man looked at me as if I were either insane or a little slow and spoke in a tone one uses with a small child.

"Ma'am, as I said there is a home game, we can't go to campus now."

I pulled him into the kitchen out of earshot of Arlan and said, "Listen, I know he can't be directly admitted to the James, but this is life threatening. Getting him to OSU is his only chance. Come on, help me out. You're in an emergency vehicle."

He continued to regard me as if I weren't terribly bright, but finally did pick up his radio to explain our situation to whoever was on the other end as they began to load Arlan on the stretcher. Ducking out the door behind it, I saw my sister come to a flying stop in front of my neighbor's house. She ran from the car looking pale and frightened.

"He broke the leg," I said as I ran to my car.

"FUCK" she yelled. "I'll be there as soon as I can!"

"Boys are in the basement, Emma's babysitting" I yelled back through the open window as I peeled out behind the ambulance.

The ER was surreal that day. By the time I convinced a police officer, who had blocked the off ramp from the highway for the football game, to let me through and made my way past security, Arlan was in a small room lying on a bed. A young female doctor came in and explained that they would take an X-ray and make a plan from there. Arlan clutched my hand, shaking from the pain. As she was getting ready to leave I requested pain meds and she suggested a high dose Tylenol. I rattled off his medical record number and asked her to please pull his file and order pain meds accordingly. She came back a few minutes later, looking grim faced and said a nurse would be in shortly with a narcotic pain shot. She had put in for an orthopedic consultation in anticipation of the X-ray results. A few minutes later the familiar X-ray machine cart came bustling down the hall and into the room. Arlan grimaced and sweat broke out on his upper lip as they positioned the film cartridge under his leg.

The portable X-ray shows an immediate picture, and I saw the technician's eyebrows knit in confusion. Having studied many pictures of Arlan's tumor by then, I stepped forward.

Knowing exactly what had changed, I pointed to an area on the X-ray. "Here's the break."

After studying it intently, he said, "Yeah, I think you're right. Are you a radiologist?"

"Nope, just his wife" I replied.

As everyone cleared the room, I pulled up a chair and sat down by Arlan's side. Having received a second injection of pain medication, he had grown quiet. I turned on the television asking if he wanted the game on. He nodded drunkenly and asked for water. Upstairs, in our usual wing of the James, I knew where most everything was kept. If Arlan needed ice water, had chapped lips or wanted a warm blanket, I simply went out and helped myself to what was needed. In the foreign world of OSU's ER, I was lost. When I ventured out to find water and call my mother-in law, I found myself in the ambulance bay and was met with dismissive waves by security as I approached the booth to try to determine how to get back.

I wandered around until I found the entrance to the ER, where I had to clear security a second time before making my way back to Arlan's room. As I approached, I noticed that several of the staff, nurses, patient assistants and cleaning people were gathered outside his door looking up at the TV in the corner of his room. I heard them groan collectively at something happening in the game. As I pushed my way through, Arlan again asked for water.

Turning to the group at the door I snapped, "Can any of you tear yourself away from the game long enough to bring him some ice water?" and then closed the door firmly.

It felt like considerable time passed before two young looking doctors entered the room. By then Arlan was in and out of wakefulness with heavy pain medication and hardly reacted. One of the doctors said he was an orthopedist and introduced the other as a resident. They had seen Arlan's X-ray and would be taking him to the operating room shortly to put a pin in the leg.

"Nope," I said immediately, shaking my head. "You can't pin his leg, the bone is too diseased."

"We do this all the time," the orthopedist assured me.

I jumped out of my seat and explained that there was no way they routinely worked on people as sick as my husband. He was in no condition to give his consent and I refused on his behalf. When I told them to page Dr. Mayerson, they responded that he was out of town, but that his partner, also an orthopedic oncologist, was in the hospital and on-call for the weekend.

"Get him" I said.

They patiently explained that the orthopedic oncologists don't come to the ER.

"Bet you he will make an exception if you call and tell him we are here and I refuse to allow you to treat my husband."

Less than a half hour later, there was another knock at the door, and a new doctor came in introducing himself as Dr. Mayerson's partner. I explained what had happened and what the other doctors wanted to do. He assured me I had done the right thing. Then, he gently explained that there was no choice at this point but to amputate. Although we had been hoping for an amputation to remove the source, I was rendered momentarily speechless at this news.

Arlan would be admitted and the amputation would happen on Wednesday when Dr. Mayerson was back. In the meantime, Arlan would be heavily medicated for pain. Although as his partner he would assist with the surgery, he wanted to wait for Dr. Mayerson, who was attending a wedding out of town. When I reminded him that Arlan had just completed chemo and was at risk for infection because his white count would be bottoming out, he responded that it would not be an issue. I was relieved to hear it and even more pleased that a room was being prepped for us on our usual floor. I could not wait to get upstairs. My sister, who had reached Alex to take over for her at the house, was en route to the hospital with our bags. We had not unpacked them yet. When transport arrived, I kissed Arlan and practically ran through the hospital to our floor.

Arlan's arrival on the floor was much like the return of a conquering hero. The nurses, assistants and the rest of team gathered by the desk and rushed around him, welcoming him back and teasing him about how they had missed him in the 24 hours he had been gone. The room sobered considerably when he was painfully moved into his hospital bed and they saw the size of his swollen thigh. Fortunately, the care team upstairs was top notch, as always, and rushed to ensure there was plenty of pain medication on order. As Arlan raised the head of the bed to make himself as comfortable as possible, we heard what sounded like a loud mechanical groan from the underside of the bed. It sounded like the bed were about to break apart.

"Uh-oh" Arlan said.

I looked over and noted that, despite the dreadful sound, he was positioned fine. "That's the least of our concerns at this point," I told him.

That night Arlan slept fitfully, fading in and out of drugged dreams. Several times he woke up screaming in pain and clutching at his leg. Although the nurses continued to dispense pain medication as often as they were able, he would be asleep one minute and then shoot bolt upright the next, shivering in bed by the time the next dose was available. This pattern continued through the next day. He was unable to get comfortable and became more and more agitated each time he tried to lower or raise the bed and it made its awful sound. Late Sunday evening, I remembered that I was supposed to have taken him in for the $5000 shot that afternoon.

I asked our nurse for the evening, a kind gentleman who had cared for Arlan several times before, if there was anything he could do, but because the dispensing clinic was outpatient only and had long since closed for the day, all he could do was make a note in the chart for the doctors the next morning.

By Tuesday morning, Arlan was nearly impossible for me to console. He was not eating or drinking and when he was awake was moaning and trembling with sweat on his brow. The days of pain had left him worn, weak and exhausted. Late that afternoon, the surgical team made its rounds and after reading his chart, the doctor in charge stated that Arlan would not be a candidate for amputation the next day.

Stunned, Arlan struggled to ask questions. The surgeon explained that because of Arlan's chemo and his white counts, he wouldn't be able to stave off an infection from such a major surgery. Amputation was out of the question. The doctor tossed around options such as a giant cast that would immobilize Arlan's lower body until his white count rebounded. I repeatedly pointed out that Dr. Mayerson's partner had assured me that wasn't an issue, but the doctor simply kept repeating the same explanation. When he and the surgical team finally left the room, Arlan's composure dissolved. His body was wracked with sobs, and he collapsed back against the bed. I tried to console him, wrapping his shoulders in an embrace while steering clear of his aching leg, but he was beyond my ability to reach; his hold of his emotions having been shattered by this development. Eventually a new pain shot allowed him to drift off into a fitful sleep.

16

Trapped in a Bad Sitcom

As soon as I was sure Arlan was asleep, I left his room and took the elevator down to where Dr. Neki and Dr. Mayerson have clinics across the hall from each other. I searched for Dr. Mayerson without success before barging into Dr. Neki's clinic. I stood in the hallway with my mind racing when I heard the comforting sound of Dr. Neki's sweet voice from the office toward the back. Without hesitation, I barged in and told him he needed to come upstairs and see Arlan as soon as possible. I explained what had happened, that we had yet to see Dr. Mayerson and that Arlan was beyond consolation. Although he had a full clinic schedule and was running behind, he promised to come see us before he left for the day and jotted Arlan's room number on a post it which he attached to his papers. He squeezed my shoulder and sent me back upstairs. I ducked my head back in and said I wanted Dr. Mayerson upstairs as well, and Dr. Neki assured me that someone from his team would hunt him down. In the elevator, I leaned against the corner, exhausted.

Late that afternoon, Dr. Neki arrived as promised and sat in a bedside chair. Arlan opened his eyes, looked at him and smiled.

Dr. Neki sighed heavily and said, "You can't have the amputation tomorrow."

As he searched for further words, the door opened and Dr. Mayerson appeared. I don't think there ever was a time I was more relieved to see someone. Just having him standing in the room was somehow comforting. Arlan's face lit up for the first time in three days, and he struggled to sit a little higher and straighter in the bed.

Dr. Mayerson leaned against the sink and asked, "What happened?"

Arlan relayed the whole story.

When he was finished, Dr. Mayerson shook his head sadly. "Sometimes this just happens; no matter how careful you are, there is a minority of patients where the bone is just too diseased to keep holding together, and it just crumbles," he explained. "It's impossible to predict who this will happen to. I'm sorry it happened to you." He also apologized on behalf of his partner, who was rather young and had simply not thought through the whole issue of how chemo and nadir would impact the situation.

After going back and forth with him for some time, Arlan reluctantly acknowledged that he was not having an amputation the next day. Honestly, I don't think he would ever have agreed, but at some point it became clear that Dr. Mayerson was not going to perform the procedure, which left Arlan no option but to accept.

Dr. Mayerson had another plan. He would take Arlan to the operating room briefly the next morning and place a steel pin through his calf which would protrude on both sides of his leg. Ropes would be affixed to the pin and a pulley system with weights would effectively pull the pieces of bone in his thigh apart. That would alleviate the sharp pain spasms caused by the jagged shards of bone rubbing together in his thigh. The procedure would pin Arlan to the bed for approximately eleven additional days until he reached nadir and the amputation could be completed.

Desperate for relief from the pain, Arlan agreed, but I struggled to understand the implications. "You are putting a foreign object in his body, won't that present a risk?"

Smiling kindly, Dr. Mayerson explained that no surgery was without risk of infection but that this was a minor, quick procedure with minimal risk. I perched on the left side of Arlan's bed trying to grasp why this was not more of a concern when I felt his hand on the back of my neck, squeezing tenderly.

Pulling me in close to him, he gently turned my head and looked me in the eye. His blue gray eyes were tired and wet as he slowly said, "It doesn't matter if the skin or tissue in my calf gets infected, baby. It doesn't matter what happens to that leg. At this point, it's coming off."

I closed my eyes briefly as the reality swam before me.

Dr. Mayerson produced an X-ray which I could have drawn from memory at this point. He cleared his throat and said, "Regarding the break, there is an issue we need to discuss."

Pointing to a large cloudy area on the picture which extended nearly all the way up the leg, he explained that what we were seeing was a bruise which was made up of contaminated blood. All the cancer cells that were once contained in the source had now been freed to roam throughout his system. As a result, he had no choice but to take the leg off all the way at the hip.

I heard the echo of my mother-law's voice when I called her on Saturday night and she said, "I only hope they don't have to go all the way to the groin." A recently retired nurse practitioner, she knew how much tougher the recovery from such a high amputation would be and how much harder Arlan would need to work to walk again.

I heard Dr. Mayerson say to Arlan, "The surgery will be scheduled just as soon as we see your numbers start to rebound. Then we will proceed with the full right hip disarticulation."

I had to have him repeat the name of the procedure twice before I got it down. Smiling kindly, Dr. Mayerson wrapped Arlan's hand in both of his, looked him right in the face and assured him that he would take care of him.

I had another thought—regarding the creaking bed and asked, "Will this be the bed he is pinned to?"

"Whatever bed they bring him down on. Why do you ask?"

I explained about the awful noise it had been making, and Arlan pointed out that in his opinion—which was an expert opinion when it came to mechanics—it was breaking.

"Remind me in the morning," Dr. Mayerson said as he stepped out of the room.

Early the next day, Arlan and I were once again waiting in the staging area for surgery. The two goofballs from our first time there were back, but I had learned a few things by then. I closed the curtains, effectively cocooning us in a safer more private space. I perched on the stool next to his bed with my forehead resting on the side rail next to his hand. It felt like years, not just days, since we got that last good night's sleep in our own bed after his release from chemo.

As is so often true in life, I had no idea that was the last night we would ever spend in our own bed together, the last time Arlan would ever be upstairs in our house. I softly hummed a tune from our children's old lullaby album to him, trying to provide a distraction from the sounds beyond the curtain while he gently stroked my hair, both of us offering comfort to one another.

At some point, a nurse came in, looked at the chart and asked Arlan what procedure he would be having that day. When he responded that he was having a pin placed, her brow furrowed. She explained that he was scheduled for a hip disarticulation. Arlan eyes became wide and I saw his blood pressure on the monitor jump.

"No, no," I quickly interceded. "That plan changed last night. Please call Dr. Mayerson."

A few minutes later, Dr. Mayerson appeared. He was not taking the leg. The surgery schedule had already been printed when he changed the orders. Everyone in the operating room knew the correct procedure. Almost immediately after he left, another doctor appeared and introduced himself as the anesthesiologist. Like the nurse, he asked Arlan a few questions, including what procedure he was having. Arlan again explained about the pin and was again met with a questioning look.

"You've got to be fucking kidding me," he said turning to me. "Get me out of here!"

"Relax," the doctor told him. "Let me find out what's going on."

"What's going on?" Arlan muttered incredulously. "What's going on is you guys are going to kill me!"

I ran my hands along Arlan's shoulders and arm comfortingly and explained as quickly as possible what had happened the night before and that Dr. Mayerson had just left, assuring us that everyone who was going to be in the OR was aware of the change.

The anesthesiologist excused himself to look into the issue and Arlan began to cry.

Grabbing my hand, he begged, "This place is like a bad sitcom. Please, don't let them take me to the operating room. I just want to go back over to the James. I'll live with the pain until my numbers come up."

Holding his hand, I poked my head out of the curtain and called to the nurse to get Dr. Mayerson back. I watched with alarm as Arlan's blood pressure continued to rise while he stared at the curtains with terrified eyes. When Dr. Mayerson arrived, we related what had happened. He explained that there is more than one anesthesiologist and guessed that it was an assistant who had visited. Although it was very cool in the room, I could see the sweat on Arlan's brow and feel his rapid heartbeat in the wrist I held in my lap. Once again, Dr. Mayerson assured Arlan that he was the only one doing the actual procedure and that he most definitely would not be amputating. Arlan finally lay back against the bed again. I pointed out how agitated he had become and asked if they couldn't give him something to calm him a little before they got started. Dr. Mayerson agreed. I reminded him that the bed had issues and that Arlan needed to be transferred to a different bed before being pinned to it.

No sooner did the curtain close behind Dr. Mayerson than Arlan began again to beg me to get him out of there. My heart was beating so hard I thought I would be able to see my sweater moving when I glanced down. I made soothing sounds and wiped his brow. The anesthesiologist came back in, this time with a syringe in his hand, and explained that he was going to give Arlan a drug which would have the dual effect of calming him and making him forget most of what had happened.

As he wiped off Arlan's IV with an alcohol swab, he looked at me and said "He's going to be asleep in just a few minutes anyway; this is a waste of perfectly good meds."

The only thing that prevented me from assaulting him was that Arlan's hand, which had been clutching mine, began to relax almost immediately. As I looked at his face, his eyes lost focus and his breathing became steady. When I looked to the base of the bed again, the offending doctor had left and orderlies had arrived. I kissed Arlan's head as they wheeled him away and swallowed the bile in my throat thinking about that doctor going into surgery with him. I comforted myself by running this mantra through my head, "I trust Dr. Mayerson, Dr. Mayerson will take care of him," as I made way to the family waiting area.

17

The Broken Bed

By early afternoon, we were back in Arlan's room at the James. He was resting comfortably with anesthesia still in his system and I was sitting quietly, relieved to see both legs still attached and grossly fascinated by the metal tube that protruded from both sides of his right calf.

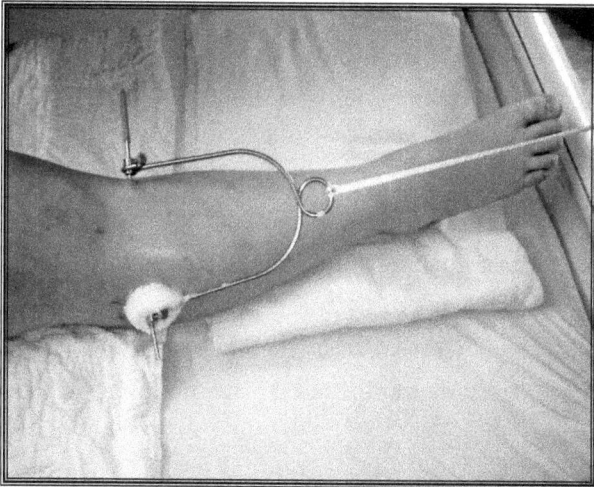

That evening when he was awake, Arlan appeared to be resting comfortably. He requested dinner, which my sister kindly and promptly ran over to us and he actually ate. He appeared to have only fuzzy memories of what had occurred in the pre-surgical area for which I felt incredibly grateful and no memory of anything from the time Dr. Mayerson came in the second time to the time he woke up with me next to him safely back in the James. His nurses, of course fussed over his leg and the pin which he assured me he couldn't feel.

His mood was amazingly good after the last several desperate days and Rebecca even brought the kids in for a short visit. Despite the relief from the leg pain and having spent much of the day sedated, Arlan was exhausted and so was I. Arlan pushed the button to lower his head and we heard the familiar mechanical groan. Clearly the bed had not been switched which Dr. Mayerson explained the next day by saying that it appeared to be working fine to him.

Over the next few days, Arlan discovered that without pain he could turn his knee a little causing a bizarre momentary protrusion in his thigh at the point of the break, which he particularly enjoyed doing as one of the nurses would lean in close to check his leg. Watching them jump and flinch, never ceased to delight Arlan and he used the parlor trick frequently. I made my usual trips back and forth to the house to see the kids each day and various friends and family spotted me at the hospital so I was able to do so. Saturday night I administered his nightly sponge bath and climbed into my own cot, listening to the groaning of his bed and then a loud crunch. Arlan immediately began to swear as he was now lying perfectly flat and the bed was no longer responding to the buttons at all.

I ran to the hall to retrieve our nurse, a young woman who had never cared for him before and she with all the nurses at the station rushed into the room. Arlan was still lying perfectly flat and let out a litany of curses damning everything from the hospital to Dr. Mayerson's ancestors while both his nurse and I tried desperately to get the head of the bed to rise again. It was definitely broken, no amount of fiddling on either of our parts made a difference. Promising to call for a repair she hurried out of the room as another more familiar nurse went to gather pillows to prop him with. The room cleared, Arlan turned to me and began to yell that he knew this was going to happen and demanding to know why he had been left in this bed. I stood there, helpless to do anything and feeling like a complete and utter failure. Intellectually I understood that he was lashing out in fear and frustration, but in that moment I was beyond tired and longed for comfort myself.

The night was endless. We were visited by various maintenance folks and even a bed technician none of whom knew how to repair the bed with him in it and no one could move him out of the bed without the orthopedic team. Arlan's nurse called for the orthopedic team about five minutes after the bed broke, but despite my begging, pleading, threatening and yelling through the night, no one came and I was continually told that they were unable to page anyone else.

As the night wore on Arlan became increasingly uncomfortable and agitated; he threw up on himself after trying repeatedly to sit up despite being pinned to the bed. He attempted to use his urinal, but could not get the angle right, spilling urine on himself, the floor and all over the bedding. His nurses and I tried frantically to make him comfortable, but after a few hours in the forced supine position with his leg pinned to the bed, his back in a continual spasm and covered in his own bodily fluids he seemed to have lost his grasp on what was happening, repeatedly indicating surprise by being stuck to the bed and asking over and over why he was in the hospital and why I was doing to this to him. I tried sitting behind him with a pillow in front of me to prop him up, but that became uncomfortable for him after about 10 minutes.

At about five the next morning, one of the nurses came in and told me that the orthopedic resident for the day would be arriving soon and would come directly to our floor to help. By this time Arlan had ceased struggling and lay in the bed whimpering intermittently.

When the door opened a short time later and a young woman stepped in I was limp with relief. The new bed was quickly brought in and with a team of two nurses, a PA, the resident and I, we moved him to the new bed while he screamed in pain. As they wheeled the broken bed away, I wanted nothing more than to kick it and strike out, but of course my anger and frustration had to wait so I could help Arlan to settle in his new bed and gathered items for his third sponge bath since the previous night. Arlan preferred not to have strangers attend to this intimate detail and I completely understood, although at that moment I felt unable to even focus on my hand as I dipped the washcloth into the basin.

Clean, in a working bed, with fresh sheets Arlan passed out from the pain, exhaustion and medication and I collapsed onto my cot. Two hours later I woke to the sound of Arlan again screaming in pain. I fought my way to the surface of consciousness to find him clutching at his leg much as he had during the days before being pinned to the bed.

"There's no tension on my leg," he cried. "I don't think this was put together right."

I ran for the nurse and while we both stared in confusion at the contraption at the bottom of his bed Arlan explained how the system should have worked and pointed out how it had been incorrectly threaded by the resident. As I gently pulled where he instructed to place tension on his leg, my anger and frustration began to bubble over. Once the pained had ebbed somewhat, I eased the weight back to the ground and the nurse went to call orthopedics back to the room.

I called my sister on my cell phone. As I poured the story of the previous night to her, Rebecca gasped in horror and urged me to demand to speak to an on-call administrator. She suggested that I go to the nursing station and request the CEO of the hospital. She told me that he would of course not be reachable (no surprise since it was early on a Sunday afternoon) but that there was absolutely, positively some administrator on call and in charge in case of a dire emergency which she assured me we were in, she also coached me to insist that Arlan's surgeon be paged even though he was currently out of town once again.

Feeling bolstered by Rebecca's words and desperate to spare him additional pain, I approached the nursing station and made my requests. The nurse who I spoke to was of course known to me and assured me that orthopedics were coming and that there was no administrator to be called. Although my brain felt fuzzy from the stress and lack of sleep of the previous night, in that moment I was so afraid that any further problems might push Arlan over the edge of sanity that I persisted. I asked who would be called if there were a natural disaster, opining that if there were a catastrophe surely there was a protocol by which someone in charge could be reached. After giving it a few moments thought, the nurse said she would page the hospital nursing director who was to her knowledge the highest ranking person in the building at the time. Satisfied I went back to Arlan's room to wait for the orthopedic resident.

I am not proud of the way I treated the young resident when she came back to Arlan's room a short time later. In a bitter and condemning tone I explained that she had failed to put his suspension together correctly and caused him additional pain and suffering and then stood over her like a mother bear protecting her young as she re-attached it. Fortunately, by then Arlan had slept enough and had sufficient pain medication to recover his faculties and was his usual kind, gentle self as he patiently explained to the resident how the suspension is supposed to work and how it was configured incorrectly. Under his watchful eye it was quickly repaired and he once again relaxed back in relief.

Shortly, a somewhat older woman appeared at the door and introduced herself as the nursing director. She kindly asked if we could go to a conference room and talk as Arlan had drifted back to sleep. I kissed him quickly and squeezed his hand before stopping at the nurses' station to tell them where I would be. I had to force myself to sit in the chair at the table. My stomach felt as if it would bubble out of my body. I wrung my hands and tensed my legs as I spoke in both the clearest and frankest manner I had to date about Arlan's condition.

"My husband is a dying man, and I am honestly afraid you people are going to kill him before the cancer ever can," I told her.

She stiffened and asked me to start at the beginning and tell her what had happened. Starting with the orthopedic team in the emergency room who wanted to take him to the operating room and pin his broken bone, I told the story in excruciating detail. As I relayed the events of the previous night, I saw tears collect in her eyes, and as I as continued to describe his experience, she began to cry openly but allowed me to finish. When I got to the end where the resident had fixed the bed, I explained that I was desperate to protect him from what felt like incompetence to me and that I was considering whether it would be possible to have him transferred to another facility but given his predicament I just didn't know.

Lost and desperate, I repeatedly said "I just don't know."

Removing her glasses and putting her pen down after taking many notes throughout my telling she rested a hand on my arm, which now sat loosely on the table in front of me cradling my head and apologized profusely for Arlan's suffering. She assured me that Arlan would be taken care of and I had done the right thing by demanding that she be called. She promised to help me investigate transport if that was what we wanted, but asked if we would first give them a chance to look into all of this and make things right.

I knew how much Arlan liked and trusted Dr. Mayerson and what incredible level of trust and affection I had for Dr. Neki, Michelle, the nurses and regular team who had cared for both of us over the months. In addition, during all my prior research I had heard good things about the James, and the proximity to home and our children was convenient. So I reluctantly agreed.

The nursing director assured me that she would begin working on this immediately and I returned to Arlan's room where I found Rebecca sitting diligent vigil by his side. I collapsed into her arms as I shared my conversation with the nursing director. Rebecca tucked me into my cot like I was a small child and brushing the hair off my forehead urged me to sleep, promising that she would watch over Arlan until I awoke.

Upon waking some time later, I found Arlan and Rebecca chatting pleasantly while watching television. I took a huge drink of the water bottle that was never far from my side trying to shake the exhaustion and dehydration. Rebecca said her goodbyes and Arlan and I sat quietly holding hands. So often during that time, I was able to focus on how much I just enjoyed being with him. Having him back to himself after the horrid toxicity event had left me with an appreciation of the gift of having him and holding his hand; sitting quietly was a joy I had learned to savor. There was a knock at our door and a distinguished looking gentleman entered the room and introduced himself as the CEO of the James. He explained that the nursing director had asked him to come and speak with us when he happened to run into her after popping by the hospital. Perhaps it is his habit to pop in to the hospital in the early evening on Sundays, but to me it seemed more likely that true to her word, she had been following up on our conversation and called him.

He asked if he could sit and if we would share with him what had happened. In uncharacteristically eager and forthright terms Arlan launched into his accounting of what had happened since breaking his leg and even before, sharing things like his frustrations with his port, his discomfort regarding the transport team while waiting for its placement and even his firm belief that no one should be forced to share rooms in a cancer hospital.

As I sat listening to him detail his concerns, filling in blanks when he turned questioningly to me, I felt overwhelmed by the journey we had taken. I noticed Arlan's jaw begin to quiver as I shared the anesthesiologists comments about the wasted drugs; a story he was hearing for the first time, and the CEO murmured that was the sort of the sort of comment that could get someone fired, shaking his head sadly. Arlan was able to detail most of our experience up to the point of the broken bed. Mercifully, he seemed unable to recall most of what had happened the previous night and as I related the events of the night Arlan became quiet and withdrawn.

Once the telling was through, the CEO smiled sadly and again extended his hand to each of us saying that he truly regretted ever hearing a story like that from his own hospital and assuring us that he would be fully investigating. He promised that we would hear from Dr. Mayerson yet that day and that Dr. Neki would be in to see us the next. He went on to outline how he would be investigating before handing us his card and encouraging me to call his office with any further concerns, vowing that we could expect far more conscientious care from that point forward. The next afternoon a volunteer from the gift shopped stopped by with a fleece blanket embroidered with the James logo and a note from the CEO again apologizing.

Although we explained that Dr. Neki and his team had nothing to do with the trauma of what had occurred, as promised, he did appear in the room to see us the next day. We enjoyed our visit with him and he stopped by frequently during the days that Arlan lay pinned in the bed. We understood that there was nothing he or his team could really do for us during that time but we treasured his kind, gentle tones, reassuring competence and the companionship of his visits. Dr. Mayerson did call that evening as well. He explained that he was out of town and would be back the following day. He said he had spoken to the resident who saw Arlan already that morning and as I railed into the phone about her incompetence and his poor judgment in leaving Arlan in the broken bed, I looked up and saw her sitting behind the nurses' station looking wide eyed and sad.

When Dr. Mayerson arrived at the hospital the next night, he also apologized for Arlan's experience. Turning to me, he strongly urged me to get out of the hospital for a while and said that often when trapped in the hospital for prolonged periods of time patients can experience a form of temporary dementia which in this case was likely unavoidable due to the need to pin him to the bed. He shared his concern that spending so much time there; I too could begin to feel these effects. I did not bother explaining that I left the hospital nearly every day to spend time with my kids and shower. Although delivered kindly and gently, I felt as if I had been slapped by Dr. Mayerson's response. To me, he seemed way too fast to dismiss the seriousness of what occurred with the challenges of prolonged hospitalization.

The other new person we met that week was Ginger. Ginger was a patient advocate who worked for the James. Renee, her boss was one of the Directors who reported to the CEO and after a series of follow up conversations with Renee, Ginger came to see us. Ginger was a woman about my age with a lovely smile and the patience of Job. She would come in to see us and focus as if there was nothing else happening in her life. Whatever we might need or mention she immediately followed up on and like so many others, she became an anticipated and beloved visitor.

18

"Bye Bye Leg"

Arlan and I anxiously awaited each day's lab reports and watched his numbers carefully for signs of nadir. As we discussed the challenges that lay ahead, one of his greatest concerns was how our children would feel seeing him without his leg. Arlan's father, who had fought diabetes most of his adult life, lost one of his feet and Arlan remembered the heartbreak and trauma of watching him go through that. Recognizing how young our own kids were and wanting them to have an easier time, Arlan proposed that they could perhaps decorate his leg before the surgery. I chimed in, suggesting we have a farewell party for his leg. Arlan, who had been busy working on his amputation humor, loved the idea.

The afternoon before his surgery, I ran out and bought an ice cream cake. He had seen one on television recently and commented that it looked good. The writing on the cake said "Bye Bye Leg," and Arlan wrote a parody of the song *Bye Bye Love* to go with it:

Bye bye leg
Bye bye bone cancer
Hello prosthesis,
Good-bye right leg good-bye.

That evening the kids crawled all over the bed. Emma did Arlan's toe nails with sparkly bright colored polish, and Jonah pressed temporary tattoos to his leg. I invited all the nurses, the doctors and passersby to enjoy some cake, and Arlan asked them to write on his leg. As I made a pass around the bed, he pulled me to him and handed me a red magic marker. He had been having nightmares that they removed the wrong leg, and I wrote in large bold red letters on his right thigh, "THIS LEG GOING"; and on his left, "THIS LEG STAYING."

Later, when I posted a picture on Facebook, Arlan and I laughed long and hard about a friend's comment, "As always, helpful to the medical staff…"

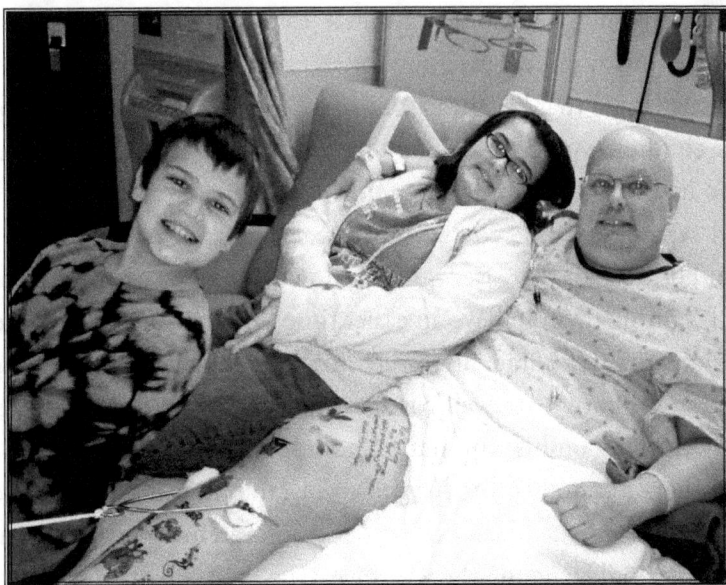

The kids left happy that night, hugging and kissing their Daddy. Emma asked if she could come to the hospital in the morning and sit with us during the surgery. Jonah decided to go to school. Following the advice of the professionals we had consulted, we allowed them each to make the choice that felt comfortable for them.

Once the room was empty and it was just us again, Arlan posted on social media, "After tomorrow I will have a 50% lower chance of stepping in dog poo."

We were laughing when a young resident knocked on the door to ask what we wanted done with the leg once it was removed.

"What are my choices" Arlan asked casually without taking his eyes of his netbook.

The young man looked back and forth from Arlan to his clipboard and explained that it could be frozen for burial later, buried now, cremated or donated.

Arlan rubbed his chin and asked, "Could I have it made into a lamp?"

The young resident's eyes widened. "Wait, what?"

"I'd like to have it made into a lamp," Arlan said with his eyes twinkling, but a serious expression on his face.

"Umm..."

"We could put a fishnet on it, and a fringed shade. It would be like a major award."

The young doctor looked slightly horrified.

I explained, "He's kidding. It's from that movie, you know, A Christmas Story—you'll shoot your eye out."

Arlan giggled as the resident shook his head.

After signing the paperwork to donate whatever tissues could be used for study and cremate the remainder, we turned off the light to rest for the day ahead.

Arlan's mom came to Ohio that night for the big surgery. She had made many previous trips, but this time she arrived with her dog in tow to stay for a while. Emma and Jonah were thrilled to have their grandmother with them, which gave Alex some needed relief. Once Arlan was safely on his way to surgery, Julie, Emma, Rebecca, Devon and I headed to the family waiting room to begin the long day of watching the board there for updates. Originally, we had been told that the surgery would take three to four hours, As we passed the five hour mark, I looked at our group, gauging by the taut faces, nervously shaking legs, and frequently shifting bodies, that we had passed the point of making idle conversation.

Emma cuddled close to my side an hour or so later when I noticed a surgeon in scrubs stepping up the ramp towards the room. It was Dr. Mayerson! I jumped to my feet and rushed toward him.

He smiled and said, "He did great."

My relief was so palpable I became lightheaded. A cheer went up from the group that had followed me and now surrounded us. I threw my arms around the doctor and then hugged each of my family in turn.

Dr. Mayerson explained that the surgery had been a success, but had taken longer than expected as the amputation was complicated by the tumor having grown additional veins to feed itself. This was apparently fairly common, but required additional care in the operating room. Arlan was minimally awake in recovery, breathing on his own, but not yet communicative. He would stay there a bit longer and then be returned directly to his room in the James. Dr. Mayerson went on to explain the plan for, and ins and outs of pain management, but I hardly heard him. As we all stood there, clutching hands and grinning at one another, the only thing I could focus on was that the source of the cancer was gone. I felt invincible and giddy.

With a celebratory air we gathered our things and decided that a treat was in order after keeping such a tough vigil and receiving such great news. We paraded downstairs to the gourmet cookie shop and bought sweet treats that we gobbled up on our way back to Arlan's room.

It was amazing how big it looked and felt without the bed in it. Having spent two weeks there already, it had become a home away from home for me, and I flopped down on my cot with my legs stretched in front of me. As I waited for Arlan's arrival, I felt I would explode with joy.

When the nurse poked in her head to say that he was on his way, I danced into the hallway. Hearing the chime of the elevator. I rushed forward to see him. The bed came into view and my smile felt frozen on my face. For six months we had anticipated the amputation and had agreed that it would be fine. None of it prepared me for how small Arlan looked on that bed, or how surreal it was to see his torso with no right leg attached. He was sitting up in the bed staring somewhat vacantly. When I rushed to his side, he turned his head, his glassy eyes staring into mine, and smiled drunkenly.

The orderly at the head of the bed needlessly offered, "He's still pretty loopy, still out of it."

Arlan reached out for me and I squeezed his hand while attempting to suppress my dismay at his disfigurement. I watched the orderlies wheel him into the room. The visitors and well-wishers, so jovial only minutes before, became silent as they encountered the horrible reality of the amputation. I turned toward the window and convulsively swallowed the bile that had risen in my throat. From the corner of my eye I saw Rebecca flee from the room and heard her barely contained sobs as she made her way into the hall. I felt Emma press against me and turned in time to see her grandmother wrap her in her arms, a figure of lonely strength watching them settle Arlan, her oldest son, in the room.

In the next few minutes that passed, I felt as if I aged years. I tried to collect myself and focus on what Arlan's nurse was telling me. He was on a morphine pump that automatically dispensed meds on a set schedule, but he could have additional pain relief every 45 minutes on demand by pushing a button. I don't know how or when everyone departed. I know I updated the blog I kept online for distant relatives, but my only focus that day and during the long night that followed was on pushing that button to keep Arlan from feeling pain. He slipped in and out of consciousness, mostly sleeping, but occasionally waking and asking for a sip of water or scratching absently as he looked down in bewilderment at the empty space once occupied by his right leg.

By late the next afternoon, Arlan began the arduous task of fighting his way back to a semblance of normal. He not only managed to pull himself up to a sitting position on the side of the bed, but stood and, holding on to a walker, took one hopping step before collapsing exhausted back into his bed.

Through that day, the next and the long nights, I never allowed myself to sleep for more than a few minutes so I could push the button as soon as Arlan was allowed pain medications. I figured that he had gone through so much suffering already that if I could alleviate some of the pain, all the better.

On the third night, the nurse came in about two in the morning and found me squatting next to the bed waiting for the timer to tick down with the button in my hand. Gently she pulled me to my feet, steered me to my cot and urged me to get some sleep. Arlan needed to feel the pain and reach for the button himself so that they could monitor how much pain he was experiencing and know how to treat him best. She asked if I had been hitting the button since surgery, I nodded reluctantly, but was relieved to see no judgment in her kind face. She only asked me again to stop. As soon as the door closed behind her, I jumped out of bed, pushed the button myself one last time and then crumbled back into my cot and fell into a troubled sleep.

As the week finished and bled into the next, Arlan slowly learned to walk again. With a utility strap wrapped around him, held firmly by physical therapists and clutching a walker, he made his way around the nurses' station while I followed behind pushing a wheelchair so he could rest as needed. Although we had done our best to prepare for the eventual loss of his leg, there were many things that we simply did not know. No one had ever mentioned that, in both men and women, it is common for the genitalia to become engorged with fluid following an amputation at the hip. Two days after surgery fluid began collecting in his groin, and his testicles enlarged to the size of grapefruits. Arlan and I were horrified when we realized that I would need to locate his penis within this swelling so that he could pee.

Similarly, we were unaware that in order to be fit with a prosthesis the wound from the amputation would need to heal. We didn't know that the wound would be gigantic, reaching from the bottom of Arlan's abdomen to his lower buttock and that his body, compromised from both the chemo and the cancer, was no longer really able to heal.

Certainly we had read about phantom pain and understood in a general and intellectual sense that it is a common phenomenon. We were ill prepared, however, for the way Arlan would physically jump or flinch when someone moved toward the bed or sat where his leg once was. He frequently complained of itching in his absent right leg, and we were both stunned when, in desperation to offer relief, I began to run my crooked fingers in a sweeping motion up and down along the area the leg once occupied, and the itching sensation subsided.

19

Going Home

As the long hospital stay continued, I found myself increasingly exhausted. Arlan was feeling the effects of nearly five weeks in the hospital, too. He was having difficulty differentiating day and night, couldn't remember when things had occurred, and shifted moods frequently. Finally, Dr. Mayerson suggested it was time to get him released, and I was shocked when physical therapists came in that day and mentioned transferring Arlan to the rehab hospital a few buildings over. Although Arlan remained quiet, he turned to me with huge, frightened eyes.

I emphatically said, "Nope, we are not doing that, I'm taking him home."

Gently, the physical therapist explained that it would be easiest for him to master the tasks of movement and self-care in the rehab hospital, and that it would be the safest place for him as well. Although I understood her position, I longed for nothing so much as to have my family together again in our home. Arlan looked at me imploringly before staring at a spot beyond the door and agreeing that perhaps the therapist made sense. I sat down next to him on the side of the bed, held his hand in mine and assured him that we had gone every step of the way together and would get through this together as well. Did he want to go to rehab? He shook his head NO. With more confidence, I again told the physical therapist I would be taking him home and asked her to send the aftercare coordinator in to assist me. I called Rebecca, and by late the next afternoon, she was supervising the delivery of all the medical equipment we needed at our house, and dear friends were coordinating the building of wheelchair ramps to the front door.

As I sat on the windowsill in the hallway, making arrangements to get Arlan home, a nurse came over and introduced herself as a member of the palliative care team. I had met several others like her before and was no longer surprised by their approach. She asked me how things had been going and nodded kindly as I shared my feelings of helplessness and fear that Arlan's wound was still seeping and might never heal. I dumped out all my frustration about living in the hospital and being away from my children, not to mention the constant pressure from relatives, friends and even strangers to remain hopeful even when things seemed to go from bad to worse.

She listened quietly before giving me the single greatest bit of advice I would receive throughout the entire cancer journey: "It is your job to speak the truth as you understand it to be. What everyone else chooses to do with that truth is up to them."

Then she strongly encouraged me to not be afraid to "read the writing on the wall" so that I could plan and make decisions accordingly and to talk with Arlan openly and honestly about it all.

That night as we lay in the hospital, with only a small night light illuminating the room, I finally gave voice to my fear.

"I'm really scared. This is just not going the way I expected. I thought you would be so much better by now."

Arlan breathed what I can only describe as a sigh of relief and said, "I'm not going to make it."

"Don't say that!"

After several minutes of silence I started again, "I understand this may no longer be a winnable fight, but please don't tell me you are just giving up. You can't give up. We have only just begun to fight."

For the first time I heard Arlan laugh bitterly and say, "I'm tired, baby. I haven't just begun to fight, I fought really hard. I don't know how much more fight I have. I'm not ready to give up, but we have to be honest: Things aren't good."

Another period of silence hung heavy in the air.

Finally he said, "We'll be married fifteen years next month."

"Yeah."

"Always meant to take that tropical trip."

Desperate to provide him something positive to focus on, I said, "You know what we should do? Let's renew our vows."

Arlan sat up and flipped on the light. "That's a great idea!"

I walked over to the bed and sat cross legged at the foot facing him, and we talked into the night to make plans to have a big family holiday followed by our renewal ceremony. We had been married the weekend following Thanksgiving. As for most couples, holidays were a dilemma, offering both joy and guilt. Which family would we celebrate with? Where would we be? The year we bought our house, we invited everyone and had a traditional holiday in our home, but since then it had been more difficult to arrange everyone's schedule and the demands of our work lives.

At some point, Arlan casually observed, "This will be my last Thanksgiving, I want it to be great."

"You don't know that!"

He looked at me for a long moment. "You're right, I don't know it, but I feel it. I'm not giving up, but let's not pretend."

I lay down next to him along his left side, and resting my head on his shoulder, clicked off the light. He held me tightly to him, running a comforting hand up and down my back.

By the end of the week, we were home again. Arlan settled in the hospital bed I had placed in front of one of the windows. It was drafty, and Arlan had usually sealed windows by this point in the season. Happily, he had been unable to do so this year, and the slight breeze provided him some comfort as he was always warm. I took up residence on the couch so that I could be nearby to spot him on trips to the bathroom in the middle of the night or to get whatever he might need. After 15 years I couldn't imagine sleeping a floor away from him anyway, so I was happy to be close by. Following such an incredibly long hospital stay, it was a huge relief for all of us to be sleeping under one roof again.

By then Arlan was nearly two months out from any chemo, and while his taste buds and general mood had improved considerably, we noted some alarming changes. Somewhere in the process, he had lost a considerable amount of his sense of touch, particularly in his hands. This seemed so odd to me. It was tough to conceive of such a thing, and yet, he had difficulty holding a pen, a fork or spoon, or stroking Emma's and Jonah's hair. His ability to concentrate had also been badly compromised. It seemed that the chemo fog or chemo brain, as it was commonly referred to around the hospital, was a real and permanent phenomenon, making it difficult for him to express himself, talk on the phone or ask for things he wanted.

Still, Arlan took all of these challenges in stride. Grateful to be back at home and to see Emma and Jonah every day, he applied himself vigorously to the physical therapy that was offered by the visiting professional three times a week. I was happy to have a nurse visiting often as well, to check his wound, which continued to seep, and address other concerns as they surfaced.

Halloween drew closer and some incredibly thoughtful anonymous neighbor was kind enough to leave pumpkins for our children on the porch. Arlan had always loved Halloween, usually walking the neighborhood with the kids. This year he clearly would not have that option, but he was adamant that he wanted to participate and would hand out candy. Arlan was the reason things remained "normal" that year. He allowed no holiday or event to be skipped. Although he had stopped expressing his hope for a cure, his hope for our family, the success of our children and our enjoyment of life remained alive and well.

The week before Halloween we visited Dr. Neki's office to determine our next steps for treatment and were dismayed to learn that Arlan's hormone levels measuring bone growth were spiking once again. This was not a shock, as he had been without chemo so long, but certainly not what we had hoped for. There was both good and bad news. While the hormone levels were discouraging, Arlan had been accepted into a clinical trial in Michigan for Sarcomas. Dr. Neki and Dr. Anderson both felt it might buy him extra time, and though it was not specific to his cancer, could provide some benefit. We were scheduled to be in Michigan on Monday, November 1, so with new possibilities on the horizon we prepared for Halloween.

Arlan came up with lots of costume ideas—peg legged pirate and shark attack victim being his favorites—but in the end sat in his wheelchair on the porch bundled in a winter coat. As kids he recognized arrived, Arlan would smile broadly and joke with them. Many appeared shocked by his appearance, said little and backed away quickly. Others seemed not to recognize him at all. Only Bella, my friend Stephanie's 3-year-old, for whom Arlan had always been a beloved uncle, squealed with joy and climbed onto his lap in the chair. Despite a few uncomfortable moments, Arlan seemed to delight in the whole event. When I finally pushed him back into the house, he returned to his bed exhausted from his exertion but with a smile on his face.

20

Not What I Had in Mind

When Arlan was first diagnosed with cancer, we discussed taking a family vacation—maybe flying with his mom to Japan to visit Scott and his family, or taking a cruise with our extended family. We had so many ideas, but as the weeks passed, it became clear that this was not likely to happen. When we heard that Arlan had been accepted to the study in Michigan, a mere three- hour drive from Columbus, we felt that we had been given a gift and decided to create a memory with our children.

Early Sunday morning I packed Arlan, the kids, his wheelchair and our luggage into the car and we headed out. We had a wonderful drive, admiring the foliage along the way and singing way too loud with the radio. I had reserved the nicest hotel I could find and had requested a room with a balcony which overlooked the lovely indoor pool and hot tub. Arlan was able to wheel himself onto the balcony to watch the kids swim. I relaxed in the hot tub; allowed the warm water and swirling bubbles to ease months of tension. When I looked up and saw Arlan sitting at the table on the balcony with his netbook open in front of him, but his eyes glued to Emma and Jonah with an expression of adoration and tenderness, I had to blink tears from my eyes.

We dressed up and enjoyed dinner, which none of us could finish, before returning happily to the room where, for the first time since his leg broke, Arlan and I were able to share a bed. We lay happily that night listening to the breathing of our children in the next bed and talking excitedly about what the trial might entail.

I woke up around eight and got Arlan's morning medications together. He was complaining of a headache and exhaustion, so I suggested he go back to sleep while I took the kids to breakfast. When we returned to the room, he was in the bathroom with the door closed. I knocked softly and asked how his headache was. He mumbled a response and I told him Emma and Jonah wanted to swim one more time. I would be on the patio if he needed me. Leaving the door to the room slightly open, I sat down at the table to fill out the paperwork for the clinical trial. After about an hour, I called down to the kids that we needed to get ready. My plan was to check out of the hotel and leave for home after Arlan's appointment. When the kids arrived, I suggested that Emma hop in the shower first.

Soon after, she came to the door yelling "Mom, come quick, Daddy won't open the bathroom door and it sounds like there is a vacuum cleaner in there!"

I ran inside thinking, "Why hadn't I checked on him?"

As I began to ease the bathroom door open, there was a solid obstruction in front of the door. I realized it was Arlan's left foot. Squatting, I reached into the crack, moved his foot and pushed the door open the rest of the way. Arlan lay naked, face down on the bathroom floor. The sound Emma had heard was his shallow, rapid breathing as his face pressed into the linoleum tiles of the floor. Kneeling next to him, I began to call his name and moved his head so he could get air more easily. His skin was cold and clammy, and he was sweating profusely.

As I attempted to rouse him, I became aware of my children and looked over my shoulder to see their terrified faces. I managed to roll Arlan over, with his head cradled in my lap and draped a towel over his groin. He briefly came to and grabbed at the walker, trying unsuccessfully to pull himself up. I gently lowered him to the floor, took the walker out of the bathroom and came back with his wheelchair, thinking that perhaps I could get him into that more easily. By then he was out cold again. I shoved the wheelchair away and called 911. Jonah was sobbing softly and Emma, sitting on the bed, was nearly hysterical.

I squatted in front of her, held her face between my hands, looked into her eyes and said, "I know you are frightened, so am I; but listen to me, Daddy is alive. A squad is on the way, and we have to get ready to get out of here."

Reaching behind me, I grabbed Jonah by the waist and pulled him into me as well.

"I need your help," I continued. "I need you to get our things together so we are ready to go when the ambulance leaves. We are going to figure out what is going on. I'm so sorry, I love you. I need your help."

Getting to my feet, I felt in my back pocket for my cell phone, its usual place, but it was not there. I found it in my purse. I had missed three calls from Arlan in the last hour! Dismay, guilt and panic washed over me as I realized he had known something was wrong and tried to get help. I opened the door to the hotel room so that the EMTs would find us. Emma and Jonah had thrown on clothes and were cramming things into bags with a speed and a thoroughness I never knew they possessed.

I have no idea how long it took for the EMTs to arrive, but at some point as I knelt on the floor cradling Arlan in my lap, I felt a hand on my shoulder and two paramedics gently moved me aside. They managed to wake him and asked him his name.

"Arlan," he replied.

But when prompted for his last name, he looked at them with confusion. They asked him where he was and the date, who I was?

"Rachel, my wife," he said with obvious relief.

"Who's this?" The paramedic indicated Emma hovering near-by. Arlan looked at her with fear and sadness and shook his head in confusion.

I quickly provided as much information about Arlan's illness and what had occurred as possible. Pulling him upright, the paramedics helped him into underwear and pajama bottoms before strapping him to a stretcher.

"We're heading to the university hospital emergency room," they said.

I gathered our bags and glanced quickly around the room. Then the children and I ran down the hall after the stretcher.

Sprinting past the front desk, I lobbed the room key to the receptionist and yelled, "Checking out!" I added our room number and quick instructions to add anything additional to the card on file; and would they please hold onto to anything we might have left in the room.

As we dashed through the front door, I heard the clerk say, "Don't worry about anything, God bless you!"

Arriving at the emergency room, the kids and I ran through the doors and saw the paramedics from the hotel filling out paperwork off to the right.

One looked up, smiled and said, "He's fully awake and acclimated now. We gave him some oxygen in the ambulance and his head cleared."

"Where is he?"

I left Emma and Jonah sitting in the waiting room looking small and frightened with huge eyes and pale faces and followed the paramedic to Arlan's room. Along the way he told me that Arlan would likely have a bad headache because he had a quite a bump on the back of the head. I nodded absently, remembering that I had noticed a lump on the back of Arlan's head a few days ago, and had made a note to mention it when next we saw Dr. Neki. I assumed that it was yet another chemo side effect or perhaps the result of one of the many and inevitable falls he had taken since losing his leg.

I found Arlan in a small room. His face broke into a relieved smile as I bustled in

"Hey, baby," he said in a scratchy voice.

"Oh my God, Arlan, what happened, are you okay?"

He explained that he had woken up when he heard the door close behind us as the kids and I headed to breakfast and been unable to get back to sleep because he had a headache. He made his way into the bathroom and, feeling a little light headed, sat on the toilet and leaned against the wall. He recalled hearing us come back to the room, but not my calling to him through the door. He figured that he fell asleep sitting there and woke at some point feeling very dizzy and strange. He tried to call for help but then decided to use his cell phone, which I had put on the tray of his walker the night before. He tried my phone several times and even left a message. The next thing he knew he was waking up in the ambulance. I asked if he remembered anything about the paramedics being in the hotel room and he shook his head. I explained as briefly as possible what had happened. He closed his eyes and tears trickled down his face as I mentioned that he had not recognized Emma.

I went to get the children. Once they were safely in the room, Arlan hugged them and joked with them. I stepped out into the hall to begin making a dent in the mountain of paperwork the hospital required and called Rebecca with our latest news. She immediately asked if she should head to Michigan.

"Yes, please," I said. "No wait, I don't know, not yet. Let's find out what we're dealing with."

I returned to the room as orderlies arrived. An MRI had been ordered for Arlan, both head and body. As they wheeled him from the room, he kissed all three of us and waved to the kids.

Really looking at my children for the first time, I noted that Jonah was dressed in jeans and an Ohio State sweatshirt. Growing up in Columbus, an Ohio State sweatshirt is perfect attire for any place or occasion, but because Michigan is the home of their bitter rivals, it was probably not the optimum apparel. Laughing, I explained to Jonah that he might get some funny looks as we headed to the cafeteria for something to drink.

We met Arlan back in the room. Shortly thereafter a woman entered and introduced herself as the chief of neurosurgery. She pulled up Arlan's MRI. A tumor had been found in his skull, which was protruding into his brain and likely caused the seizure. She speculated that it was likely osteosarcoma metastases and would have to come out. Arlan, who over the past several months had turned the pallor of parchment paper, became even paler. I nodded to the doctor and walked out of the room to call Dr. Neki's office.

When Kay, his assistant, came on the line I explained what the MRI had shown and held the line while she tracked down Dr. Neki. A short time later, his familiar voice came through the phone. He agreed that the tumor had to be removed as radiation was extremely ineffective against osteosarcomas. He had not taken an MRI of Arlan's head before we left because metastasis to the head or brain is extremely rare in osteosarcomas, occurring in less than 2% of all cases. I shared that they wanted to take Arlan to surgery as soon as possible and that I was terrified of being so far from home without having his full history at hand. Dr. Neki empathized with my fears and assured me that Arlan was in extremely capable hands. While I understood the need for surgery, I wanted to bring him home for it. Dr. Neki gave me his cell phone number with instructions to call him when I had a plan for transportation. He would begin making calls to assemble a team for Arlan, and took the names of the doctors in Michigan we had spoken to. I was to give them his cell phone number and not to work through the hospital's office staff at this point. In his quiet, gentle manner he reassured me that together we would get Arlan home.

I called Rebecca and filled her in on the latest developments.

"Is it safe?" she asked.

"I don't know yet, I don't know." Hearing her chuckle softly, I asked, "What's funny?"

"You wanted to make a memory for the kids."

"This is not exactly what I had in mind," I said and joined in, laughing.

I returned to the room in time to see a volunteer come in with a University of Michigan football. He gave it to Jonah. The neurologist wanted him to have a proper memento of Michigan, given his chosen attire. The volunteer took him and Emma back to the waiting room by way of the cafeteria for a snack, and I faced Arlan. I shared my fear about him having surgery in Michigan. He immediately agreed. He only wanted to be safely back at the James on his usual floor with his own nurses.

"What I wouldn't give to see Michelle come through that door," he told me.

As with so many major decisions in our lives and marriage, we were immediately on the same page. Having solidified our front, I had the ER doctor paged.

When he returned, we explained our decision. He suggested that mercy flights were very expensive, but possible, and he would put in a call to the airline. He explained that he had given Arlan some meds to prevent further seizures and he should be stable. Then he announced in a very somber tone that there was something else we needed to discuss. Bracing ourselves for the worst, we held on tight to each other's hands as the doctor called up the computer in the room.

Breathing as if he was carrying a big weight, he said, "We need to talk about what we found in your lungs."

Letting out a huge breath of relief, Arlan laughed and said, "You scared me there. That's old news."

I explained that we knew there were more than thirty nodes in Arlan's lungs, and that there was little connected healthy lung tissue left. The doctor raised his brows as if surprised and amazed by our lack of panic. Then he suggested that, based on the advanced state of disease in Arlan's lungs, he thought it best to return him to Ohio under medical supervision. I again called Rebecca who was already on her way to Michigan with Devon, her husband. For the next few hours, plans were made, changed, and changed again, as the doctors in Michigan and Dr. Neki's team worked together to get Arlan safely home.

21

Homeward Bound

It was a little like a comedy routine. I called Rebecca and Devon to turn them around after being told I could drive Arlan home. Fifteen minutes later I called again when that plan was nixed and the final decision was made to send him by ambulance. Fortunately, they had anticipated getting another call and simply stopped for a snack rather than heading back. So it felt like only a few minutes had passed when the doors to the emergency room opened and Rebecca and Devon rushed in. I leaned against the wall for support; my knees felt weak. Jonah and Emma launched themselves at their aunt and uncle—their ride home. When we all made it back to Arlan's room, his arm trembled as he reached out to pull Rebecca close.

By the time he was loaded into the ambulance that would take him home, it had become dark outside. Glancing at my phone, I realized that it was well after 9 p.m. As I settled in my seat next to the driver, my cell phone rang. It was Dr. Neki. A room would be ready for Arlan when we arrived. I could hear the fatigue in his voice as Dr. Neki assured me that he would be awake and that I could call at any time, if I needed him. We drove through the night, stopping by the side of the road twice as Arlan became ill vomiting. We waited while nausea medication took effect and his stomach settled. Fortunately, he slept for most of the trip.

When we arrived at the OSU Hospital, we were ushered into the emergency room despite my insistence that Dr. Neki had made prior arrangements for Arlan's admission to the James. By then it was after one in the morning, and I chose not to call him as Arlan was moved into a room in the emergency department.

The paramedics from Michigan who had transported us safely to Ohio stood around making small talk while they waited for clearance to begin their long trip home.

"Be careful," I told them. "I know you're tired, stay awake."

Arlan piped up that he was tired, too.

The paramedic who had ridden in the back, caring for him during the trip, patted his arm and kidded, "You're tired? You slept most of the way."

"Nope," Arlan told him. "I was awake the whole time."

The paramedic winked at me as Arlan drifted back to sleep.

Once again, I had a lump in my throat as the elevator doors opened on our floor and the night nurses rushed to greet us and help with bags. Apparently, they had been briefed by Dr. Neki's team and had been waiting for us all evening. One of our favorite nurses was on that night. She hugged me tight and led me to our room where a cot was all made up for me. The next day I learned that she had gone to three different floors to find it, determined that I would have a place to sleep.

The first of the new doctors to make an appearance was the neurologist, a middle aged transplant from New York with a great smile and a heavy Brooklyn accent. He explained that the tumor was growing from the skull into the small cavity that divides the hemispheres of the brain and was essentially a ticking time bomb.

"In some ways, although I can't tell you exactly what happened up there, this is the best case scenario," he told us. "Now we know it's there and we can start treating it before it gets bigger."

The neurosurgeon would, of course, do his best to get all or as much of the tumor as possible. After that, Arlan would then undergo a series of radiation treatments for good measure.

When I questioned this—we had been told so many times that radiation is ineffective for osteosarcoma—he explained that Arlan had exceeded the lifetime dose of the chemo that is most effective. The others did not really cross the brain membrane.

When we met the neurosurgeon, Dr. Elder, he told us that Arlan needed some time before the operation so that the blood thinners I injected him with twice a day to prevent additional blood clots could clear his system. Two full weeks would be ideal, but there was enough urgency to justify proceeding the following week. Prescribing yet another, higher level of pain medication, he released Arlan until the surgery.

Arriving back at the house was not the triumphant return we had planned when we left for Michigan, but we were relieved nonetheless. For the rest of that week Arlan was very quiet. I frequently walked in on him fully awake, sitting silently while one of the bizarre reality shows he had become interested in was playing, but paying no attention to the television.

When I asked him if he was okay or what he was thinking about, he would sometimes say nothing. At other times he would respond with things like, "I'm going to make a manual so you'll know how to take care of the house." Or, "You're going to have to stay home with the kids for a while."

Although I would listen to these snippets, I consistently reminded him to think positively and to remain focused on having as much time as possible. We no longer pretended that he was going to survive, but I continued to hold onto the belief that there was no immediate, real danger.

22

Brain Tumors

The day before his operation, Arlan called me to his bed in the early morning hours and told me that he didn't want any more chemo. Inside, I wanted to scream, but I calmly lay down next to him in his bed and told him I understood and that the decision was his. He nodded and I heard him sniffle in the dark. After several minutes he began to speak again. He encouraged me to go back to school and finish my master's degree. I agreed that I had always intended to do so and probably could find an online program. Arlan thought that made sense because after his being home with Emma and Jonah for all their school years, it would be hard for them if they were suddenly alone. He talked about insurance money and how it should be spent. He encouraged me to pay off any debt we had and not to worry about medical bills.

In the dark of that early morning, I understood that Arlan had accepted that he was going to die, but it was not something I was ready to face.

After kissing Emma and Jonah, Arlan and I left for the hospital early the next morning. Although Emma wanted to come with us again, I remembered the horror of Arlan returning to the room following the amputation and did not let her. Promising to call her as soon as we knew anything, I reminded her that Arlan wouldn't even be scheduled to come out of surgery before her school day was over. Leaving my mother-in-law, Julie, to get the children off to school, Arlan and I drove in silence to the hospital where Rebecca and Devon met us in the lobby.

As the four of us waited in his half of the room for him to be taken to the staging area, we struggled between forced small talk and uncomfortable silence. Finally transport arrived and Arlan whispered quietly to Rebecca-I later learned that he had asked her to take care of me, not to let me wallow in grief or be lonely, and watch over our children before kissing her Devon and Julie, who had joined us. As we headed downstairs, I was surprised when we turned a different way on the surgical floor. Just before taking Arlan through a series of doors and an airlock, the transport driver stopped and said it was time for me to head to the waiting area.

"No," I told him. "I go with him until he goes into the OR."

Arlan who had been holding my hand as I walked beside his bed, closed his eyes and shook his head. "I don't think I can do this," he said.

A nurse came and asked what was going on. I quickly explained. She patted Arlan's hand and told him to hang on; she and I would meet him on the other side of the doors.

She steered me quickly into a small room. Reaching into a drawer, she pulled out a giant yellow suit that looked like an oversized set of pajamas with a hood. She instructed me how to put it on and had me cover my hair with a cap before putting up the hood on the suit and handed me cloth slippers to cover my shoes. Looking not unlike a giant yellow Oompa Loompa, I followed her out through a different door and past the airlock into the bay where Arlan waited.

"Wow," he commented. "Look at you!"

"I'm a vision," I said.

An older Asian woman entered the room and introduced herself as the chief of anesthesiology. She had a heavy accent and I had to concentrate hard to understand her. I could see from Arlan's expression that he could not follow her. As she spoke, I repeated her words, close to Arlan's ear.

She ran through the usual litany of questions and then, putting her clipboard aside, said, "Your lungs are in very bad shape; we will monitor you carefully."

Then she left the room.

I kissed Arlan several times, and we clasped hands, staring at one another without speaking.

Finally, I whispered, "I'll see you on the flip side."

Arlan responded, "I love you." Watching Arlan being wheeled down that hallway was perhaps the most frightening moment of my life. The atmosphere prior to this surgery was much more somber than the others, and this from a patient who had a leg amputation. I didn't need him to tell me that he feared he would not survive the operation. In the time since our return from Michigan, he had been focused forward, not on himself. Although my emotional strength was failing, Arlan's was strong.

I stripped out of my paper pajamas and made my way from the pre-surgical bay to the family waiting area. I leaned my head against the wall and took a moment to channel all my love and strength to Arlan. My fear felt like a heavy weight pushing on my shoulders, making it difficult to take a full breath. In the family room, the tension was almost a physical presence, taking up space and sucking the air from around us. We sat in silence. The only sound was my mother-in law's knitting needles clacking.

Hours went by before we received a phone call from the operating room. All was well, but Arlan was still in surgery. Finally, the board updated that he was headed to recovery. We cautiously clasped each other's hands as we waited to hear from the surgeon. Eventually, Dr. Elder arrived looking tired and serious. He led us to a small, private waiting room off the main area and explained that they had taken as much of the tumor as they were able to, but because of the size and location, they simply could not remove it all. He believed he got enough to buy Arlan some time, but was vague about what that meant. Arlan would have another MRI in the next eight hours, which would give a better picture of what was left, and radiation would be started soon. He shared that they had had "a couple of scary minutes" getting Arlan off the ventilator, but that he was breathing on his own and would remain in recovery for some time before being moved to the surgical intensive care unit (SICU) for 24 hours. After accepting our thanks, he held my hand for a few minutes, patted my mother in law on the shoulder and left us.

We sat in the family waiting room until we received the call that Arlan was awake and responsive. Breathing huge sighs of relief, we hugged and kissed Arlan's Mom who headed home to be with Emma and Jonah.

Rebecca, Devon and I made our way to the SICU waiting room, where a sign in the lobby invited us to check in with the staff and make ourselves comfortable. People sat in clusters everywhere, huddled under blankets, stretched out in makeshift beds, playing cards, mindlessly nibbling on snacks or staring absently at televisions. Signs posted around the room explained that visiting hours were strictly enforced, and I realized in dismay that the final visitation of the night would likely end before Arlan was brought upstairs. I checked with the desk, and the nurse confirmed that he was still in post-op recovery, but promised I would have a chance to see him whenever he was brought up. Devon offered to run to the cafeteria, or even go out to pick up dinner, as it had gotten late and we had skipped lunch, but my stomach turned at the thought of food, and Rebecca and I declined.

Finally at around 8:30, the receptionist told me Arlan was on his way up. Soon we were standing in a glass room—with windows to the outside along two walls and a floor to ceiling window to the nursing station along a third—as Arlan was wheeled in. He opened his eyes and looked at us. He told us with a scratchy throated voice that his head hurt. He told me he had been a little nauseous downstairs and had continually asked for me.

A male nurse came in, looked him over carefully, and offered to let us stay a few minutes. I asked if I could stay the night if I promised to sit on the window sill and stay out of the way, but he shook his head and explained that for the well-being of the patients in the SICU, who were among the sickest in the hospital, it was important to make sure they had their rest and visiting hours were strictly enforced. He gave me his name and the phone number and assured me he would be caring only for Arlan and one other patient through the night and I could call anytime. Arlan nodded and said he understood; we should all get some rest.

Rebecca and Devon said their goodbyes and left with the nurse so Arlan and I could say goodnight in private.

For the first time in the seven months of Arlan's battle, I would have to leave him alone, and I knew he was hurting. While I struggled to maintain a smile and calm demeanor, inside I felt I was crumbling. I was panicked at the thought of leaving him like this, and my pain for having to do so felt almost unbearable. I was so frightened.

Standing by the side of his bed, I tried to focus on Arlan as he spoke, but found that I couldn't clearly hear him. His face was going in and out of focus. I began to sweat and knew I was going to faint. Leaning close, I kissed Arlan quickly. I told him I loved him and I would be back at 5:30 in the morning when visiting hours began. He should ask the nurse to call me, if he needed me. I promised to call and check on him.

Using the walls for support, I made my way out of the room and back to the waiting area. I pushed past Rebecca and Devon into the ladies room to splash water on my face. I managed to lock the door before I slipped to my knees. I must have fainted for a minute because the next thing I remember is Rebecca knocking on the door. I pulled myself up to the sink and ran the cold water over my wrists before letting her into the room. Rebecca looked at me and pushed me down onto the toilet. She held a paper towel under the running water in the sink and put it on my neck.

"You need to eat something," she said. "There's nothing more you can do here."

23

The SICU

After finally getting home to kiss my children and eating a quick dinner, I crawled into my makeshift bed on the couch waiting for 4:00 a.m. to come. Arriving back at the SICU well before dawn the next morning, I noted many of the same visitors lying quietly in groups around the darkened room. At 5:30 a nurse came out and asked us to form a line. When I stepped up and stated the name of the patient I wished to see, I was told that he was getting an MRI. His nurse came out and told me Arlan had had a great night and was doing well. They had taken him about an hour ago and he promised to call me as soon as Arlan got back.

I sat in the waiting area watching the clock anxiously as families went back to their loved ones and came out again. At 7 a.m., when visiting hours were over until 10, I asked again when Arlan might be back. The nurse buzzed me through saying that he had just been returned to his room and that I could spend time with him for a few minutes even though visiting hours had ended. Gratefully, I followed him back and found Arlan lying in his bed, clutching a little blue bag. He smiled when I came in and reached for me with his other hand.

"How'd you do last night?" I asked.

He shrugged and told me he had thrown up down in MRI. "The people down there are really great. They took care of me."

"Haven't you been taken care of up here?"

He shrugged again and said, "I'm so cold. I have been sick on and off all night and my head hurts."

"Did you tell your nurse?"

"I haven't really seen him much."

I went into the hall, found the heated blankets and covered him up. Then I went to the sink, wetted a washcloth and wiped his face.

"Better," Arlan breathed before lying back and closing his eyes.

I sat on the window sill trying to make sense of what he had said. Was it his perception that the nurse hadn't been around or had he really been alone? I became aware of two people sitting at the nurses' station talking about their preferred ice cream spot in town. They debated it for about 10 minutes in loud, jovial tones. Each time they mentioned a particular parlor, they broke into laughter. Arlan shifted uncomfortably in the bed, once moaning that his head hurt. The conversation outside the room ended when a nurse approached and mentioned her patient whom she described as "so crazy." Her description of the specifics of the accident that had brought him to the hospital and his confusion each time he woke up was also met with hysterical laughter. Seeing Arlan clearly disturbed by the sound, I felt my anger boiling in my stomach.

I had been told that I could not sit with him through the night because rest was so important for him, yet the staff members clearly had no regard for how their behavior was disturbing him. A short while later, I heard Arlan's nurse talking with a new nurse on the floor. Waving a hand in our direction, he told her that Arlan had had an uneventful night and should be moved at some point to a step down unit for patients needing less intensive care. Then he launched into a lengthy discussion of how far he lives from the hospital and how long it takes him to get home. I turned my head away in disgust and noticed that the machine that should have been attached to Arlan's remaining leg to prevent blood clots was sitting on the other window sill. It was basically an air pump which attached through hoses to a boot. Placed over Arlan's leg and foot, it gave a small massage every few minutes to keep his blood flowing. Following his amputation, he wore it for almost two weeks, and I couldn't figure out why it was sitting unattached on the windowsill.

Finally, just before 8:30, a young man came in, identifying himself as a surgical resident. I immediately expressed my concerns about the machine. He responded that, yes, it should probably be attached to Arlan, but it wasn't a big deal as it was mostly a concern for those with a history of blood clots. When I told him that Arlan had exactly such a history, he nervously moved to send in the nurse to set it up. A few minutes later the nurse who had been chatting with last night's nurse about his long drive home entered the room. She told me I would have to go back to the waiting room as visiting hours were over until 10.

"Not until I know for sure that you will be taking care of my husband," I responded

"That's what I'm doing" she said.

I pointed out that the people at the nurses' stations were disturbing him, that his leg was not attached to the machine, and that I had found him nauseous, cold and in pain.

"I just got here," she said.

I reminded her that she had been here at least 45 minutes and had not been in to see Arlan at all. "I will be back at 10," I alerted her and left.

On my way out of the SICU, I saw that the door with the sign "Nursing Manager" was open. I knocked, walked in and sat down in front of a woman who introduced herself as "Debbie."

She listened quietly and eventually said, "Well, you have to understand, people talk to each other in their work space; it is simply human nature. I will look into your concerns and let you know what I find out."

As I headed back to the waiting area, I felt the knot in my stomach begin to burn and started to panic thinking about Arlan back in that room, cold, sick and in pain. I found the business card of Dr. Calugiuiri, the CEO of the James, in my purse and called his office. I explained to his secretary who I was, that Arlan was in the SICU at the Medical Center and that I felt desperate because of the treatment he was receiving. She told me that the CEO was out of town, but promised to make sure that help was on the way.

As I waited, watching the clock, a young woman arrived, introduced herself as a patient advocate and asked which patient I was here to see. I told her. Hearing the tension in my voice, she asked if everything was all right. I told her that it was not, but that I had called Dr. Calugiuri's office for assistance. She asked if I would like to step into a private room and discuss anything. Frustrated and angry, I said quite loudly that I did not want to step into a private room, that everyone waiting there has loved ones in the SICU and had a right to know that they were not being cared for and were being laughed about. At that point, she walked away.

A short time later, Debbie appeared. She explained that it had taken some time to get in touch with last night's nurse because of the distance of his commute, but the machine had been connected to Arlan's leg all night. He had simply forgotten to hook it back up when Arlan returned from his MRI.

Debbie shrugged and held out both hands palm up. "He simply forgot," she said. "Is there anything else I can help you with?"

I shook my head and walked away from her in disgust.

At 9:50 I went to the door leading into the SCIU and hovered there until 10 when the woman at the desk pushed the button to buzz me in. I hurried to Arlan's bedside where I found him more awake and wearing his boot with the machine humming intermittently.

I leaned down to kiss him and asked how he was doing.

"Not so good."

He had woken up several times throughout the night, sick or in pain, and been unable to get help. He had kept pushing the button on the bed, but no one came. I tried pushing the button myself and searched for the remote unit that was usually clipped to the side of his bed. It operated the TV, adjusted the bed and also had a call button. I found it attached to the wall, two or three feet behind the bed; there was no chance he could ever have reached it.

"I'm so sorry, baby," I said, running my hand over his brow. "I called Calugiuri's office; someone is coming."

He shuddered. Putting his hand to his head, he repeated that his head hurt.

I went to the wall, pushed the button, walked into the hall and began yelling Debbie's name.

When she poked her head out of one of the rooms, I said, "He is still in pain. I need you to help him."

"I'll be there as soon as I can," she replied.

I returned to Arlan's room and burst into tears. Fortunately, Ginger entered right behind me.

Collapsing into her arms, I sobbed "Please get him out of here. PLEASE!"

I described what had happened as Debbie and Arlan's nurse came in and asked him to rate his pain. Debbie stated that they had been in the room repeatedly and that Arlan had not complained of pain, which he quickly denied. Ginger turned toward the wall and made a call on her cell phone while I walked to the end of the bed and rested my hand on Arlan's leg.

"I'm not leaving you again unless security pulls me out," I assured him.

I heard the machine begin to pump air, but could not feel the boot inflating. When Ginger hung up, I motioned her over and told her that the boot was still not hooked up correctly. She rested her hand on it for two cycles and shook her head—it never inflated.

Her phone rang and she answered quickly. Turning back to us, she said, "Transport is on the way. We are moving you to the James."

My relief was so great, that I could not contain my tears.

Ginger got us settled in the James on the 10th floor, which is reserved for neurosurgery patients, and left with my eternal gratitude. Julie had arrived at the hospital after seeing Emma and Jonah off to school, and I filled her in on the events of the morning as the nurses carefully and efficiently switched out the machine and got Arlan's boot inflating. They dispensed pain meds and made sure anything we might need was on hand. Their competence, compassion and kindness was a balm to my frightened and weary soul. Arlan fell almost immediately into a deep sleep. Julie and I exchanged smiles of relief as we sat quietly watching him rest.

I left the hospital briefly to pick up Emma and Jonah from school. I answered their questions as best I could and assured them they could visit Arlan soon. Then I rushed back to the hospital to trade places with Julie.

24

There Is No Plan

Arlan woke up a short time after Julie left and looked around the room in confusion.

Gazing out the window at a nearby construction project he said, "This is not good!"

"What's not good? What's wrong?"

Looking around again, Arlan said, "Blue walls, blue everywhere; they are boxing us in, trapping us. Make them stop, they need to stop building."

With growing alarm, I pushed the button for the nurse and tried to soothe him, assuring him that all was well. While I could not stop the construction, it was simply the building of the new hospital and had nothing to do with us.

When his nurse came in, I quickly repeated what Arlan had said as he looked around the room with obvious worry. The nurse approached his bed, checked his vitals, and asked about pain. Arlan responded that his headache was bad again, but his greater concern was that he appeared to be trapped inside the movie *Avatar*.

"I understand," she said in a calm and steady voice. She maintained eye contact with him for some time before taking a serious look around. "Let me see what I can do about that construction," she said as she walked toward the window. She quickly lowered the blinds, closing them completely.

As soon as the window was completely blocked Arlan lay back against the bed once more. "Better," he breathed. "That was close."

The nurse left and returned shortly with his next pain shot and he slipped back into sleep. Then she turned to me and explained that he was still feeling the effects of the anesthesia and may not have been fully awake. I sat back amazed and disturbed by the exchange.

Later that evening there was a light knock on the door and Dr. Elder popped his head in. I was relieved to see him, anxious to share what had happened the previous night and that morning.

He listened with a puzzled frown and at some point interrupted, "That all sounds awful, but I need to tell you what the MRI showed."

My heart sank as I realized that whatever I was about to hear would not be good. Glancing at Arlan's sleeping form, Dr. Elder suggested that I follow him to his office around the corner. I did, and he explained that there was a larger margin of cancerous tumor still in his brain than they had hoped, and that a second tumor was developing as well which had not been visible the previous week. This told them two things: the disease was very active, and Arlan was growing tumors at an alarming rate.

I asked, "What is the plan now?"

Dr. Elder sighed, removed his glasses and rubbed his forehead. "There is no plan" he said softly.

"You won't take this tumor out also?"

"Can't," he responded.

While in theory they could keep taking Arlan back into surgery and remove the tumors as they developed, it was doubtful that they could keep up with them. In addition, although this was a significant issue, it was not the primary challenge.

He looked me straight in the eye and said, "Operating on your husband, I had some of the scariest few minutes of my career. We really thought we weren't going to get him off the ventilator. I can't imagine he would be cleared by anesthesia again. He is no longer a surgical candidate."

We sat in silence as I absorbed this information.

"What does that really mean?" I finally asked.

Rubbing his forehead again, Dr. Elder leaned forward and explained that Arlan would have radiation to try to control his pain and keep the tumors as small as possible, but they were essentially helpless to prevent new ones. He believed there would be more.

"How much time do we have?"

Dr. Elder shrugged helplessly. "It's nearly impossible to say, but it is likely not long."

Despite all that had occurred I was stunned. I felt as if I had been punched.

Dr. Elder went on to explain that he needed Arlan to concentrate on getting his strength back. He was concerned that this news might devastate his ability to do so. Perhaps we should hold off sharing it with him for a few days so he could heal a little. I numbly nodded my agreement. I made my way back to Arlan's room, shivering, and settled into the side chair for the night.

I drifted in and out of sleep through that long night, wrestling with what I should do. As much as I had tried to encourage and support Arlan, I believed to the core of my being in his right to make his own decisions, as long as he was able, and I believed that to do so he needed all the information. I was overwhelmed with the guilt and responsibility of keeping this secret.

As the days passed, Arlan again fought his way back, eventually learning to walk for the second time in as many months. I noticed that he was easily moved to anger now and frequently frustrated. I hoped that getting him out of the hospital and back to the house might help. The day he was scheduled to be released, I nervously awaited Dr. Elder's arrival. We had decided that we would share all the news with Arlan that day. When the doctor hadn't appeared by early afternoon, I closed the door and faced Arlan. As clearly and concisely as possible I told him what I knew and why I had decided to keep it from him. Arlan smiled sadly. He said he understood and, slipping on his head phones, said he needed a few minutes. I picked up my e-reader and sat quietly in the corner staring at the screen, listening to the steady in and out of Arlan's breath.

25

Renewing Our Vows

We decided to conduct the ceremony to renew our vows in our own home. It was clear by now that we would not be having a large gathering, but Arlan's siblings and their families were headed to Ohio, and my siblings and their families were coming as well. Rebecca, whose marriage, I had officiated after obtaining a license on the Internet, seemed the obvious choice to perform the ceremony. Without her assistance and support we could not have survived the trials of these many months. Arlan shared with me that he could not have felt closer to her if she were his sister rather than mine.

For three days it was just Arlan and me at the house all day while the kids were in school. He slept much of that time, but when he was awake, his netbook was open in front of him. Awake or asleep, he constantly had on the television—with one odd reality show after another chronicling life that Arlan could no longer live.

As he made his way out of the bathroom late one morning—with me clutching tightly to the strap around his chest since he was not yet cleared to walk on his own—he stopped and stared at the door between the house and the garage. When we moved into our house years ago, Arlan, or "Safety Boy" as I liked to call him, was upset that the door into the garage did not lock and was not a standard, fortified exterior door, just a wooden hollow core. He had gone out to the hardware store and purchased an appropriate door, which had sat waiting the last seven years in our garage to be framed and hung.

Now Arlan turned to me and said, "I hate that fucking door. I want the new door installed."

"Okay."

"Promise me."

"I'll call someone today."

He turned to me with a sorrowful look and said, "No, not now; after. Please just promise me that it will be replaced."

I bowed my head in grief and nodded.

Arlan's Mom, brother Scott and his daughters arrived in Columbus a few days before Thanksgiving. Scott's wife Beth would join us after she finished attending training that the Navy required. Arlan was thrilled to have them with us, and his face shone with joy when his young nieces climbed onto his left leg and snuggled with him as he read a story. While Emma and Jonah were still in school, I indulged in the rare opportunity for a few hours away from home. I took the girls to breakfast and shopping, knowing that Arlan was safe with his brother. Scott asked a slew of thoughtful questions about various aspects of his brother's care. I demonstrated how to hold the strap to help Arlan keep his balance, and we discussed when to let him try walking on his own and when to offer assistance. I had not realized until these conversations how much Arlan had deteriorated over the past few months.

Since Scott and his girls stayed at our house, he and I met in the early morning for coffee. Sitting at my kitchen table, we discussed our fears about what was happening, our common love for Arlan and many other things, finally laying the foundation of a real, close and warm relationship.

When he asked me how aware I thought Arlan was of what was happening, I answered honestly, "Arlan knows that he is dying. I think he understands and accepts it more than anyone. If you ask him about it, he will talk about it openly."

Like Rebecca, Scott was unfailingly supportive, offering kindness, love and compassion even as his own heart was breaking.

Although we were delighted to have our family together for the holiday, having so many people around quickly became overwhelming. Arlan woke up on Thanksgiving morning in tremendous pain. I offered all possible medication to get his headache under control and tried to keep the eleven young kids in the house as quiet as possible while he winced each time he moved. We dimmed the lights in the family room where he lay in his bed, encouraged the kids to play elsewhere, and tiptoed around as much as possible. My step-mother and sisters brought the meal they had prepared and served us.

It never even occurred to me to try to help with food preparation that Thanksgiving, beyond making an apple pie with the kids—at Arlan's insistence—which I had done every year since Emma was born. I put a plate of Arlan's favorites together and then sat on the floor next to his bed. He pushed the food around without eating.

At some point I stood in the kitchen with Beth and reflected, "I know this will be his last Thanksgiving. I hate that he is hurting; that it is turning out like this."

After what felt like hours, with all of us smiling excessively and trying to make small talk, I finally gently suggested that Arlan was tired and needed to rest. Looking tremendously relieved, everyone filed out as quickly as they had arrived.

Despite the somber tones of the holiday, Arlan encouraged me to go midnight shopping with Emma as in past years. Promising that she would be awake and in the room with him, Julie pushed Arlan's sister, Carla, me and our girls out the door for a few hours of fun. I bought a number of bargain items, including a sweater for Arlan to wear to our ceremony, and rushed home in time to dispense the next set of medication even though I knew full well that my mother-in-law would do so in my absence. Everyone slept late the next day, Arlan slept nearly all day. I worried that we would need to cancel the small ceremony, we had planned for the next afternoon, but Arlan insisted that it would be fine.

We had decided to not only renew our vows, but exchange rings with our children as well, to give them something to hold on to that carried the message that our love for them and one another was a circle without end. Rebecca's best friend, a jeweler, generously provided rings for the four of us. They were beautiful titanium bands engraved in Hebrew to read, "Family is a home for the soul forever and ever."

Our actual anniversary fell the day after Thanksgiving that year, but knowing Arlan would need a day to rest between the holiday and the simple ceremony, we had scheduled for Saturday.

The morning of the ceremony Arlan woke in good spirits. He mentioned his headache but assured me it was better than it had been and that he was excited. I set up his bath items and clothes in the downstairs bathroom and went upstairs to shower and get dressed while Scott helped Arlan get ready. I sat in my bedroom trying to hide the circles under my eyes with concealer when the kids came in with scrubbed faces looking clean, neat and happy. I knew in that moment that we had made the right choice to carry through and was once again humbled by Arlan's ability and willingness to act selflessly for our well-being. His hope for me and the children to move forward in a healthy, loving way had become his central focus.

Returning to the family room, I found Arlan fresh-faced and beaming with pride as he sat in his recliner. When Rebecca and the rest of my family hurried in, we gathered in front of the television, which was blessedly turned off, and had a short, bittersweet ceremony. Arlan stood up with the help of his walker for the five minutes of the ceremony, and though his gaze was tender and loving, I could see the fine sheen of perspiration on his brow and the tremor in his arm as he gripped the metal handle.

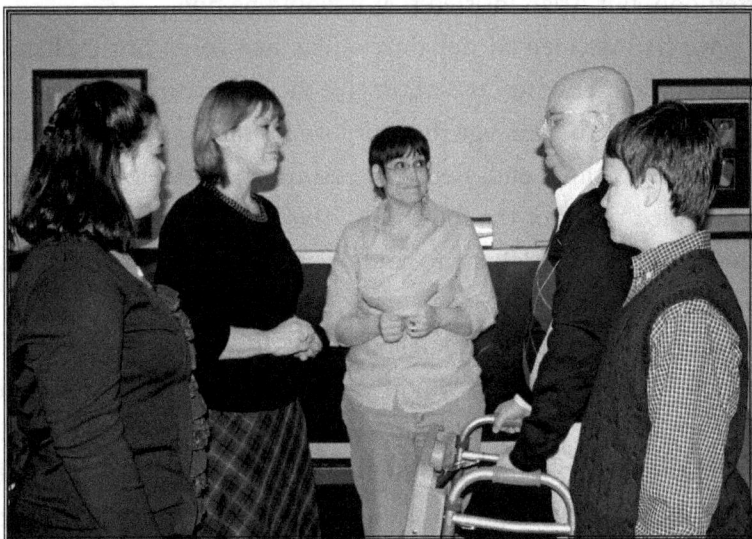

As soon as the ceremony was complete I guided him to the nearest chair where Emma, Jonah and I surrounded him, climbing onto his lap and occupying the arms of the chair to have pictures snapped. Eventually we moved Arlan to the couch and took photos of the various family groupings before breaking out the beautiful cupcakes Rebecca had provided. After nearly two hours, the extended family left, and Arlan put his pajama bottoms back on and lay in his bed with a content smile. It was one of the happiest days we enjoyed in a long time.

26

Pneumonia

But it took its toll.

Arlan barely managed to wake up long enough to say his good-byes the next morning as everyone but Scott left for home. Scott was staying an extra ten days and moved into the guest room. The house felt very quiet once everyone had departed. Seeing how exhausted Arlan was, Scott, the kids and I tiptoed around the family room, mostly letting him rest.

On Monday, Emma and Jonah went back to school and Arlan, Scott and I quickly fell into a routine. Scott and I took turns spending time sitting with Arlan, talking quietly, or watching inane television programs between his naps and nurses' visits. Arlan seemed unable to shake the exhaustion from the holiday. I worried about the tumors growing in his head.

We were scheduled to see Dr. Neki the following Wednesday. Early that morning, as Arlan and I were settling back into bed following one of many trips to the restroom, he called me to him. Snuggling in close to share some of his body heat, I lay against him in the small bed.

Arlan rubbed my back gently and said, "I'm not going back into the hospital; I mean it, no more chemo."

I lay there quietly for several minutes, then kissed him gently. "I understand," I said. "I will support your decision no matter what."

Arlan kissed me several times and I could feel that he was hoping to make love. This surprised me after so long. When he was first diagnosed, both Arlan and I were so preoccupied with fear and processing information that we were not even thinking about sex; and when chemo started, it almost immediately became a moot point. As is common for many men, Arlan experienced impotence following the first round. Although we were able to be intimate in other ways through much of the treatment, making love was no longer possible. But now, after he had been away from chemo for a substantial length of time, he wanted to.

Having slept little and rarely more than two hours at a time since I could not remember when, I was thoroughly exhausted. "Honey," I told him gently, "I need to be up with the kids in just a few hours."

"It's okay," he said.

"I love you" I told him.

I lay there thinking that I wasn't even sure of the logistics of intimacy at this point, considering his still unhealed wound. I silently reasoned that when Emma and Jonah were in school and Scott back in Japan, we would be alone in the house, and there would be time to make love again. But that never happened. To this day it is perhaps my greatest regret. More than three years later I continue to agonize over the choice I made that night.

Taking care of Arlan had become my fulltime and primary job, and I had become good at it. Knowing that being fussed over drove him crazy much of the time, I had developed covert ways of doing so. Monitoring his temperature was a necessary step, so I had become adept at doing so by kissing his head. I made it a habit as I wheeled him to the car for appointments. That morning, however, I gathered our bags and sundries while Scott wheeled Arlan out and stowed the wheelchair in the car. As we waited for

Dr. Neki in the clinic, I noticed that Arlan looked flushed and was sweating; but he was warm so much of the time that I dismissed it as normal. When our turn came, we sat in the exam room while the nurse took his vitals. I was shocked and horrified when she announced that his temperature was over 103. I jumped up, kissed his head and realized he was burning up.

Immediately Arlan said "I don't want to be admitted." He turned to me with tears in his eyes and begged me to keep him out of the hospital.

I promised to try. He, Scott and I sat quietly and anxiously waiting for Dr. Neki. He joined us a short time later, saying he had called upstairs to have a room prepared. Both Scott and I suggested that we could care for Arlan at home in whatever way was needed, but Dr. Neki insisted that he needed to be admitted. He suspected pneumonia. Once this was cleared up, we could talk about next steps for chemotherapy.

I immediately piped up, "No more chemo."

"Then the lung tumors will keep growing," Dr. Neki said sadly.

Arlan was admitted a short time later and taken for a chest X-ray. I was not surprised when it came back inconclusive. The doctors started him on high dose antibiotics anyway and ordered a chest CT for a better look.

By early the next morning, Arlan's color was a little better and he seemed less sleepy. Chad, our nurse practitioner, stopped in. The chest CT had come back showing evidence of pneumonia. It had been tricky to see behind the tumors in his lungs. When he offered to show me, Scott perked up. Having seen pictures of Arlan's lungs many times by then, I stepped back so that Scott could have a better view. The images on the computer looked like an obstacle course of cloudy barriers and narrow spaces, and Scott turned to me in confusion, asking what he was seeing. Numb to the images after so many months, I responded that the cloudy things were tumors. Scott stiffened in shock as he realized how truly bad things were.

While it was one thing to say how much cancer was in Arlan's lungs, it was another to actually see it. I noted with some dismay that the tumors did appear to have grown since my last look. We went back to Arlan's room and Scott approached the bed where his brother slept with a look of such grief and love that I slipped quietly outside to give them a few minutes privacy. When I returned, Scott suggested that he had been thinking it might be good to get Arlan a small video recorder which he could use from his bed to journal or record messages. This seemed like a wonderful idea. With the first night of Hanukkah only a day away, I picked one up when I left to see Emma and Jonah.

By the third day of that hospital stay, Arlan had perked up considerably. His temperature came down and stayed down. We were surprised when there was a knock at the door and Dr. Neki, the neurologist and two women we did not know entered the room. Dr. Neki introduced them as palliative care nurses, and Arlan, Scott and I exchanged uncomfortable glances. Dr. Neki again went over the lung CT, confirming that there had been significant growth since the last scan. We listened tensely as we tried to interpret what this might mean.

When Arlan suggested that he was considering maybe one more round of chemo, Dr. Neki sighed. "I will keep going as long as you want me to." he told him. "At best maybe it will buy a few days, but those are more days in the hospital."

Scott asked, "You don't think it's worth trying, do you?"

Dr. Neki repeated what had become a familiar refrain. "If it were my brother, I would say no. Go home, enjoy the time you have."

"Listen carefully to what he is saying," the palliative care nurse told us. "He is no longer talking months or weeks. He is talking days."

I looked at Arlan in the bed. He reached for my hand and rubbed his thumb against it. Smiling sadly, he said, "Here I thought it was the brain that was going to get me, but I guess it has been the lungs all along."

Seeing him sitting there with decent color, awake and interacting with us, it seemed that it could not be true, even as I signed the paperwork to enroll him in hospice. Dr. Neki and the neurologist agreed that we should move forward with radiation to control the pain in Arlan's head, but made clear that we had past the point of hoping for any real reduction of his brain tumors. Standing up, Dr. Neki embraced Arlan and then Scott and me in turn. He hugged me warmly and whispered that I had done well. I should keep hold of his number and call any time we needed him. We made an appointment for a social worker to come to the house the next day to help us talk to Emma and Jonah about the decision we had made. Exchanging hugs and kisses with the staff, who had become our family and lifeline over the last eight months, I wheeled Arlan out of the hospital and down to the car Scott had warmed up to take him home.

We arrived back at the house just before sundown. Leaving Scott, Emma and Jonah to help Arlan get settled, I hurried into the kitchen and in a flurry began to make potato pancakes, apple sauce and soup so that we could celebrate the first night of Hanukkah. Arlan was in great spirits and his eyes shone with love for us all as we lit the candles and sang together. He loved the video camera and rubbed his hands over it excited to have a new gadget. We gave Emma and Jonah small gifts that I had tucked away long ago. When we opened a package from one of our out-of-state relatives, to my horror I found it to contain gifts for the children and me, but not for Arlan, and I threw the box across the room in fury. Scott followed me into the kitchen, trying to soothe me, reminding me it was likely a result of not knowing what to send, and that it was the day's news compounding my feelings. I got myself together, and we went back to the table and played a game with the children, laughing and talking into the evening.

27

Hospice

The hospice social worker arrived right on schedule the next day. Arlan was sitting up in his bed, while Emma and I sat in chairs, and Scott and Jonah were on the couch. Occupying the space between Jonah and the armrest was Molly, our Great Dane. She sat there tall and quiet lending support with her head high and her massive chest puffed out as if to say, "Lean on me. I'm here for you."

We explained to Emma and Jonah what hospice was: We were no longer actively fighting the disease but had chosen to try to manage the symptoms. Arlan shared that he would get progressively sicker, and that we didn't know how long it might be, but that he was going to die. This was the first time we had spoken so frankly with them and both of our children recoiled slightly at the news. I struggled to remain calm on the surface, but inside I was trembling. I was not ready to face this myself, yet I was asking my children to look at the ugly reality without any clear answers. My mind raced with questions, desperate to know how much time we had and frantic to find a way to make it last longer.

We explained in terms as simple and clear as possible what was happening. What we couldn't tell them was why or how quickly things would progress. Although I witnessed it, the courage it must have taken for Arlan to have this conversation is beyond my ability to imagine. Not only was he facing his own mortality with clarity, but comforting all of us in the process. He spoke to the children about how his death would mean that he would no longer be physically present, but assured them that they would never truly be alone as he would always be with them, nearby, loving us all.

After much agonizing, Scott finally made the decision to head back to Japan. I know this was a difficult choice for him, and I sat for many hours at the table with him while he struggled between his love and obligation to his family and his desire to be with Arlan. I know the two brothers talked a good deal, for which I am truly grateful. I do not know what was said, but whatever it was; it allowed Scott to reach the decision to head home and left Arlan with a sense of peace.

The following week was "Donuts with Dad" at Jonah's elementary school. We were fortunate to live in an affluent suburban district and had long been active in our school community. Arlan attended every school function, field trip, and event, and he was determined to make this one as well. I was very nervous about the idea of Arlan, recently released from the hospital after a bout with pneumonia and with no immune system, sitting in a cafeteria full of young children. He shrugged off my concern, seemingly no longer worried about risks and focused solely on making sure that Jonah knew he was there for him. No sacrifice was too great for that.

I called Tyler, the principal, who had provided tremendous support to us and our children during this trying time. He arranged for us to sit in a different room, isolated from the other kids and parents. When the day arrived, we pulled up at the school several minutes after the event had started, and with the help of Jonah's Intervention Specialist Jessica, I hustled Arlan safely into the designated room. Arlan and Jonah beamed in matching smiles as I snapped pictures of them there together.

Later that afternoon I found Arlan in his bed with the video camera set up in front of him.

"Making some movies?" I asked.

"Just playing around, trying to figure out how this works. Actually, I'm making a list of all the video messages I want to make."

The thought occurred to me that he might be better served to just make the videos rather than the list as I joined him on the bed. He looked at me with a very serious expression on his face.

"I am thinking about making a video for whoever you are with next," he told me.

"What?" I exclaimed, making a face and starting to get up. "Don't say things like that!"

"No, listen to me." He reached out to put a restraining hand on my arm. "I don't want you to be alone. You should find someone else and be happy. I want you to be happy, and I want whoever is lucky enough to have you next to know how special you are, and to know how much I love you. I want them to appreciate the gift they are getting and to cherish you."

My throat felt thick and full, I simply could not form words. I sat there for several minutes stroking his arm before finally saying "I love you baby, I don't want anyone else. I haven't always been the wife you deserved, but I have always loved you."

He held his palm to my face and said "I love you."

Then he leaned back and closed his eyes.

When Emma came in from school a short time later, he called out, "Is that you, Pookie Dookie? Come lay down with me." Pulling her down next to him in the bed, he wrapped her in his arms.

For the next few days, Arlan slept a great deal, but was alert and engaged in between times. I watched him with the kids, frequently calling them back to his bed for extra hugs and kisses, holding them to cuddle and whispering in their ears. I saw him listening to music and watching television and thought to myself that we had made the right choice. He seemed peaceful and happy, but also intensely focused on his interactions with me and the children, as if wanting to make sure that he was giving all that he had.

I knew he was experiencing considerable pain, and I consulted with Dr. Anderson. I e-mailed him the most recent update, he responded briefly, "No more chemo, radiation for pain management only, time now is very short." We visited the radiation lab on a Friday for Arlan to be fitted for the mask he would wear during his treatment. The prototypical geek, he was excited to learn about the process they would use to pinpoint where the radiation would go and protect the rest of his body. I smiled when he came back to me in the waiting room, gushing about how cool the process was and showing me the video he had made of his mask.

On the ride home late that morning, he sighed wearily and said, "I've been thinking, I don't think I want to be cremated."

We had previously discussed death and shared very similar sensibilities about the body being nothing more than a shell, always agreeing that we cared little for what choices the other made regarding interment, as we "wouldn't be around to see it." We had both expressed a mild preference for cremation without doing much concrete thinking about it. At our young age, it had never seemed terribly urgent. Now Arlan was clearly telling me that he wanted a different choice.

"I want the kids to have a place to go, a place to grieve so their lives aren't consumed with it," he explained.

"Okay", I said, swallowing convulsively.

28

The Beginning of the End

I called Rebecca that same afternoon and shared our conversation. "I can't believe I am really thinking about this," I told her "It feels surreal."

"You don't belong to a temple," she reminded me. "Do you want me to call a few?"

I did not. Thinking back to the early days of our marriage, I asked if she remembered a rabbi named Lauren. She had worked at the temple that we all once belonged to. We became quite close, and our friendship had led to us and our husbands enjoying some dinners together, celebrating our kid's birthdays and participating in various other social activities together. Lauren had long since moved away and we had lost touch, as young families often do.

I said to Rebecca, "I wish I knew how to reach Lauren. She is the only religious official I could even imagine calling."

"I understand," Rebecca replied.

With usual efficiency, she took over the task of finding a funeral home and identifying a grave site.

Meanwhile, we awaited the arrival of Arlan's aunts and uncles. Growing up in rural Pennsylvania, Arlan had always been very close to his extended family. He and the children had enjoyed vacations with aunts, uncles and cousins each summer until he became ill. Although I had remained in constant communication with his family through our online blog and they had sent count-less cards and notes, he had not seen any of them since then. When his mom had mentioned during one of her many calls that her sisters, brother and their spouses wanted to come to see us, Arlan beamed with joy.

They arrived the day of Arlan's radiology appointment. They came in two cars, so that Julie could stay on with us for a few days. Arlan was exhausted and in pain, and although I continued to dis-pense medications as often as possible, we could not get ahead of it. By the time Julie called to say they were turning onto the street, Arlan had finally fallen into a fitful sleep. I was loathe to disturb him, so I waited on the front porch and went out to the arrivals to explain the situation. These were some of the people who loved Arlan best in the world and, despite a seven hour drive, they un-derstood. I took Julie's bags and she tiptoed into the room and kissed Arlan as he slept. I recommended a nearby restaurant where they could grab a quick bite.

By the time they came back to the house, Arlan was awake again and sitting up in bed. He hugged and kissed each of them as they came in, closing his eyes and smiling as they embraced him. I stretched out next to him on his bed, as I often did when the room was full, and listened to him and his uncle engage in a lively conver-sation. They stayed for an hour or so and then left for their motel. As his Mom walked them to the door, I saw Arlan rest his head in his hand crying softly. I rubbed his back and wiped away his tears.

The next morning Rebecca called bright and early and said, "I found her!"

"Found who?"

"Rabbi Lauren, I found her!"

After we'd hung up the previous day she had begun searching and had discovered that Lauren was living in Atlanta.

"She's going to come, and she's going to call you," she told me.

Sure enough, that afternoon, Lauren called. We had as lovely a conversation as was possible under the circumstances—talking first about Arlan, then catching up generally on our lives, and agreeing to keep in close touch as things progressed. Lauren assured me she could be here as soon as she was needed.

Arlan enjoyed another short visit with his aunts and uncles that day. Again, I stretched out next to him during the visit, but jumped up quickly when Arlan complained of discomfort as I laid my head on his shoulder.

"Not on my chest," he said, rubbing at his shoulder. "I hurt today."

It was the first time that had happened. Afraid of hurting him again, I hovered around the end of his bed. Arlan exchanged quiet words with each of his relatives, in particular his Aunt Rose, as they said their goodbyes and headed home to Pennsylvania.

Arlan seemed profoundly weary that day. I offered to get his wheelchair as he sat up to make his way into the bathroom, brush his teeth and get ready for bed. He waved me away and used his walker. I was standing nearby when he called for me, and I rushed to the bathroom, where he was clinging to the sink. Gasping for air, he asked me to get the chair, and I brought it back quickly so he could collapse down into it. I got him back in bed as he continued to fight for breath. Desperate to help, I brought him fresh water, raised the head of the bed and massaged his back, but nothing worked. I called the hospice number and waited anxiously for a return call. I assured him that I would work on getting him oxygen when we returned to the hospital for radiation on Monday if hospice couldn't get it sooner.

When the nurse returned my call, she said she would work on getting the oxygen, but that it probably wouldn't help because

Arlan's lungs were shutting down and too diseased to process it effectively. She suggested we play music, leave the television on, and provide other distractions that might help him relax. She would bring over a few additional medicines to keep him as comfortable as possible. I went back to the family room where Arlan had again fallen into a fitful sleep.

The hospice nurse arrived early the next morning. After fighting for air all night, Arlan was exhausted and struggled to sit up. She examined him and produced a urinal for him to use instead of trying to get up. I reminded her that he was scheduled for his second radiation treatment in the morning, but she didn't think he would be well enough to go. She suggested I let him rest and see how he did the next day. Before leaving, she produced some paperwork. It was a Do-Not-Resuscitate form, known as a DNR. She reminded me that the most basic principle of the hospice program was to allow a peaceful and natural transition from life to death, with no intervention in the body's process. I stared at the form for some time until my mother-in-law came in.

She looked at it over my shoulder, put her arm around me, and smiling sadly, said, "It's time. You need to sign it."

I was overwhelmed by this woman, her love for her child and her ability to choose his need to be released from suffering over her own to cling to him. Her courage inspired me. Taking a deep breath, I quickly signed the form.

29

Goodnight, My Love

It was a quiet afternoon and evening, I struggled to get Arlan to swallow each dose of medication and coaxed him to take small sips of water. Rebecca and some close friends came and went. Rebecca had scheduled an appointment for us the next evening at a funeral home. I nodded woodenly, hearing without listening to the details.

Arlan's hospice nurse arrived with the oxygen she had promised. As she had predicted, it made no difference, even at the highest concentration. Arlan had not left his bed that day and although he attempted to use his urinal, he was not able to produce any fluid. The nurse said that it was because his bodily functions were probably shutting down. His body no longer needed food or water, and it was uncomfortable for him to ingest them.

"What does this mean?" I asked.

"He is beginning the process of dying" she explained.

I rubbed my arms which felt suddenly cold as ice. When I asked if the kids should be at school, she patted my arm and assured me that nothing was likely imminent.

Rebecca came by that evening to take me to the funeral home. She joined Emma, Jonah and me. We were sitting on the couch, piled under blankets because of the bracing temperature in the house—it was turned down because Arlan sweated and complained of heat.

When I told the kids dinner was ready, Arlan, who appeared to be sleeping, piped up, "I want dinner."

"You do?" I asked in disbelief.

"Yeah," he responded without opening his eyes.

I went to the kitchen and placed a tiny bit of food in the middle of a small dessert plate. I took it to him on a tray and laid it gently in front of him. He raised his head slightly and I moved back toward the couch.

No sooner had I sat down than Arlan asked, "Are you done yet?"

"Me?" I responded.

"Yes, are you done eating?"

"Yep, are you?"

"Yes," he exclaimed with a huge sigh.

Rebecca and I looked at each other. He never actually looked at the plate, let alone touched it.

"Might as well get ready for bed," he told us.

Rebecca and I exchanged amused glances as he had done nothing but sleep for the past two days without leaving his bed.

When I told Emma and Jonah I was going out with Rebecca to run a few errands, Julie knew exactly where we were heading and hugged me as I got ready to leave. I leaned over to kiss Arlan goodbye, while she suggested I turn on the TV in case he woke up and wanted to watch. In my heart, I knew that he was done with television, but I went ahead and turned it on.

"Maybe bring him a frozen coke," Julie told me.

"I'll try," I said, knowing that he wouldn't drink it and likely wouldn't even know it was there.

At the funeral home the director met with us and we began the heart wrenching process of making choices for a funeral. It felt like a surreal, dreamlike trance as we made selections walking in a room filled with coffins.

After much agonizing, I decided it was time to visit the Dublin Cemetery and look at the few available plots, since Arlan had been so adamant and excited about moving to this suburb, and I wanted him to be close to where we lived.

I returned home to find Arlan exactly as I had left him. I went upstairs to read with Emma and Jonah and tucked them in, kissing them each and offering extra hugs and cuddling. The next morning they came in to kiss Arlan goodbye as they headed out to school. He sighed wearily as if the effort to even speak to them was simply too much. I called Rebecca and asked her to go to the cemetery for me. I was afraid to leave him even for a minute. She purchased a single plot with another next to it. She wasn't able to bring herself to buy the second one, knowing it was for me. I understood and made a mental note to contact the cemetery about it at some point.

Julie, who had been scheduled to leave for home that day, decided to stay on another night. I spoke to Scott on the telephone and expressed my concerns about her driving back home emotionally and physically exhausted. I was also afraid she might not make it back if things changed quickly. Julie and Scott spoke for some time and when she hung up, she told me she would be staying for the foreseeable future.

The following morning Arlan was coming off another shaky night. When I woke him for his morning meds and to say goodbye to Emma and Jonah, he seemed almost unable to lift his head, but he managed to whisper his love to each. I dropped the kids at school grateful that their friends would provide some distraction from what was happening at home. Back at the house, I tried to dispense Arlan's morning meds. When he finally opened his mouth to my cajoling, I dropped all the pills in and tipped his cup up, reasoning it would be easiest to get them down all at once. He managed to swallow them and shook his finger at me as if I were a naughty child before collapsing back against his bed.

When the hospice nurse arrived a few hours later, she examined Arlan and asked to speak to me in the dining room.

"Something's changed," she told me. It was difficult to characterize exactly, but she suggested that it was time to pick Emma and Jonah up from school and gather family around us.

"Is this it?" I asked, my head swimming.

"I can't say for sure," she said. "It is so difficult to know, but something has changed, he is slipping away. I would let the schools know the kids will not be back till the New Year."

I sunk down into Arlan's office chair, needing to think about how to deliver such news to my children. I dialed Scott and Beth's number in Japan. It was the middle of the night there, but Beth answered on the first ring. My voice broke as I delivered the news. Scott got on the phone assuring me that he would be heading to the airport as soon as he could arrange a flight.

"I'll tell him," I promised. "I'll let Arlan know you are coming."

I tried to practice what I might say to my children. I decided to pick Jonah up first. Tyler Wolfe, the principal, stepped out of his office when he heard my voice.

Wringing my hands I said, "I need Jonah. Hospice said it was time to bring him home."

Several people hugged me, I don't know how many. I was so numb that it was almost as if I were watching the scene play out without really participating.

When Jonah appeared, I held him in my arms and told him, "Daddy is really struggling. His nurse thinks it's time for you to be home, for us all to be together."

Jonah's eyes filled with tears and he followed me out of the office.

At Emma's school, I gave my name to the school secretary and explained that I needed to take Emma home. Her guidance counselor stepped into the office and asked if Arlan was still with us. I nodded and explained hospice had sent me.

Then Emma rushed into the office, with her coat on already, dragging her things behind her. "Mommy?" The unspoken question shimmered in her eyes, tears already flowing down her cheeks "It's okay sweetie," I told her, taking her in my arms. "Nothing's changed since I dropped you off, but it won't be too long."

Jonah hugged his sister from behind and I shifted so that both my children were in my arms. I wanted to absorb their pain, ease their fears and shield them from what was coming. I imagined that when the kids and I returned to the house Arlan would wake up and have some sort of meaningful and perhaps dramatic interaction with us. The reality couldn't have been further from that fantasy. We did all file into his room, and he did half wake up mumbling something as Emma and Jonah spoke to him, turning toward the sounds of their voices. Finding him more or less unchanged, they curled up under blankets on the couch with books and video games.

His nurse and I spoke softly in the kitchen. "It may be time to transition him to IV meds," she told me.

I was greatly relieved given the challenge of getting Arlan to swallow anything, but desperate to help him control the pain.

The nurse called a team to come to the house, help access his port and bring the supplies that we would need for the next few days to keep Arlan comfortable. They would show me how to push the meds through his port. Having watched it done countless times at the hospital, I felt confident I could handle it. Soon, a team of hospice nurses were sitting in my dining room, pre-filling and labeling tubes of medication. After carefully explaining each vial, what it was for and how to dispense it, they accessed his port. Arlan woke briefly when we removed his t-shirt and I explained that we were going to access his port so he wouldn't have to take pills.

"Yeah, good, good," he muttered.

I was surprised that he did not flinch when the needle went into the port, but not surprised when a second attempt was needed to get it properly accessed.

Standing over his bed, one of the nurses called to him asking if he was in pain.

"Pain? No, no pain," he grunted.

"Arlan, how bad is the pain?" I asked.

"Yeah, yeah, pain," he responded as his hand moved absently toward his head.

Under the watchful eye of the nursing team, I dispensed the first vial of medication. Arlan appeared to settle into the bed as it emptied from the vial. I was tremendously comforted by feeling that I had eased his pain. After a few minutes with his breathing still labored and gasping, I noted that he was still moving restlessly. Based on his knit brows, tense face and intermittent shifting, the nurse concluded that he was still in pain. She suggested I wait another few minutes and push a second dose if he did not appear more relaxed. After about fifteen minutes I pushed it into his system and watched as his brow smoothed and his muscles relaxed.

"Oh My God," I said to Julie, "did I hurt him?"

"No" she assured me. "But he may have slipped into a coma."

I rushed into the dining room where the hospice team sat. "Come quick." I beckoned.

They hurried into the room as Julie called to Arlan with no response.

The nurses tried unsuccessfully to elicit a response themselves. "Call him, call his name," they told me.

I did and he turned his head in my direction, making a small sound.

"Try again," they urged, and I did, several times with no additional response.

"It's hard to say" they said. "He may or may not be in coma, but he has definitely slipped into an altered state of consciousness."

"Will he wake back up?"

"Impossible to say, but he can probably still hear you. Now is the time if you have something to say."

They explained that he would likely leave us within the next few days. Emma and Jonah had tears streaming down their faces as they kissed Arlan and told them they loved him. Julie leaned over and holding his face in her hands said something to him as well. Standing behind him at the head of his bed, I felt the tears pouring down my cheeks as I kissed his forehead, neck and face.

Holding his head in my hands, I leaned close to his ear and said softly, "Arlan, you are the love of my life and I will miss you every day for the rest of my life. Watching you struggle has been the hardest thing I have ever done, but you fought well, you put up a good fight. I am so proud of you; you are so brave. When you're ready, you let go. Don't worry about anything else, just let go. I got this baby, I got it."

I kissed his head and face repeatedly and stood there for a long time. I finally realized that the phone was ringing and went to answer it. It was Scott with flight arrangements. I shared the change in Arlan's status and that we didn't really know how long he would remain like this or if he would wake up.

Julie came into the kitchen and we held each other for several minutes before we both began to make family calls. Carla and Aunt Rose were already planning to leave for Columbus early the next morning. Alex came over to provide support and help care for Emma and Jonah. Rebecca and my younger sister Sarah were already there having arrived at some point. My mother made flight arrangements for the next morning.

As I went to settle back under the blanket on the chair, Julie put her hand on my shoulder and suggested I turn up the heat.

"But Arlan is so hot," I said.

"He's past the point of hot or cold now," she assured me.

I did as she told me and went to my computer. I sat down in front of it and turned to Julie, "You know what just occurred to me?" I asked. "You know what we need? I can't believe I didn't think of this before. We need a better lung surgeon!"

"No my dear," she said and gently led me back to the couch.

Before leaving for the night, Arlan's nurse explained the various medications and times they should be dispensed again. Then she handed me a small pill bottle. I could place one of the pills inside his mouth under his tongue to help control the rattling phlegm in his breath, which is commonly referred to as the "death rattle." It didn't bother Arlan, but if it disturbed us, dispensing the pill would simply make it more comfortable to sit in the room with him. Having sat with my father on the night of his death, I was familiar with the phenomena and unalarmed. I was shocked, however, that I had somehow missed the fact that Arlan, in addition to the rapid, shallow, gasping breaths since the weekend, was also emitting these sounds. Putting the pill bottle on the counter I explained to the group that Arlan hated taking meds and as the rattling was bothersome to us and not him, I was not going to dispense them. Everyone nodded in understanding.

Emotionally exhausted and physically weary, my sisters left and we settled down for the long night. Jonah decided to sleep in the basement, as he often did when frightened or worried, and Alex gathered bedding and followed him there to keep him company. Emma asked if she could stay in the family room with Arlan and I made up my couch bed for her and settled into Arlan's recliner. Molly kept us company, waking occasionally from whatever dreams dogs have. I drifted in and out of sleep for short periods. When I awoke for good, I listened carefully as Arlan gasped and fought for air. Emma winced and cried out a few times throughout the long night when there was a particularly loud or raw sounding rattle, but she closed her eyes again when I stroked her hair and reminded her that it was not bothering her Daddy.

Around six the next morning Julie gave up trying to sleep or pretending to sleep and joined Emma, Arlan and me in the family room. By eight Alex and Jonah emerged from the basement.

I looked at the kids sitting on the couch with Alex and at Molly resting at their feet, and said "Well, we made it through the night."

"Yep," Alex agreed.

Emma and Jonah dragged their spoons through cereal bowls while Julie made and poured coffee that we didn't drink. Aunt Rose called to say she and Carla were almost ready to leave. At nine I dispensed additional pain medication as the log indicated and collapsed back into my recliner while Julie checked e-mail sitting in the chair next to me.

I studied Arlan for some time.

Suddenly, Molly stood up. With canine grace she walked to Arlan's bedside and began to whine and cry. She was inconsolable. Finding no immediate cause for her distress, I tried to pull her away thinking she needed to go out or perhaps wanted breakfast. Finally she went back to her kennel and lay down, whimpering softly. I glanced at the clock, which now read 9:10 and I fell back into my chair. I closed my eyes before it registered that I no longer heard Arlan's rapid, shallow breathing.

I jumped up and screamed "Mom!"

As Julie and Emma approached the bed, I heard the sounds of Jonah and Alex running to the room as if from far away.

I felt as if my legs could not support me and anguish flooded through my body. "No, no," I screamed, oblivious to anything other than Arlan's still body lying in front of me.

Time passed and I knew with certainty that his short, cruel fight had ended.

The rest of the day was a blur. The house filled with people. I know I called hospice and they arranged for Arlan to be transported to the funeral home and his bed to be removed from the house. I vacillated from sobbing to feeling completely numb. I know I sent a text to the large group who had been supporting us. "He's gone," was all it read because really there was nothing more to say. I went on the blog I had maintained and posted that Arlan had passed. My mother, Aunt Rose and Carla arrived at some point. I know that Rebecca, my mother and I went to the funeral home and finalized the arrangements. I sat for hours on the bench in my kitchen, in my recliner, just sat. Sometime late that evening, Scott arrived. Clinging to him in my front hall, I apologized over and over, knowing that he had come so far and that Arlan had been unable to hang on and wait for him. To my horror, I learned that he had checked his phone between flights when he stopped over in California and made the remainder of the trip after reading on the blog that his brother had died.

30

You're in My Soul

When Arlan and I got married, our first dance was to the Rod Stewart song *You're in My Heart*, a familiar, funky ballad we both loved. I remember Arlan holding me in his arms that day, and the entire venue melting away as we moved around the floor while he sang softly in my ear. When the chorus played, all of our bridal party, our families and other assorted guests who had gathered around the dance floor, chimed in. In the wedding video, you can see us both jump a little when that happened. We were so enchanted with one another at that moment, but I remember feeling as if I were surrounded by pure love. Over the years we uttered those words to one another countless times. It was more than our song; it was our pledge.

Some women cry gracefully, others look lovely in their grief. I was neither and managed to get through the next several days with puffy eyes and a swollen face. I have little to no memory of the actual funeral or when various family members said their good-byes and returned to their respective homes. Emma, Jonah and I rang in the New Year with more than a few tears. Eventually I realized that it was time to return upstairs to my own room.

The first month was indescribably difficult; the first six months, a nightmare; the first year, a terrible and seemingly endless blur of anguish and pain. We got through it somehow, my kids and I. I found that the whole experience had changed me unalterably, but the core of me was still there.

Arlan had prepared us well. I would like to say that it is my indomitable strength and cocky grit that propelled our family forward, but that would be a lie. The truth is that by careful words and painful conversations, Arlan had implanted in us a belief that we would not just survive but thrive. For our children the adjustment to losing their father, as well as the changes in me, were difficult. I recall one of them telling me that it felt as if when they lost Arlan, they lost me as well. We talked often, cried together and apart, and held each other up as we found our way to a new normal.

Our lives have become a testament to Arlan's efforts to move us forward and each of our accomplishments is like a promise kept. When Arlan was sick, he read about "Relay for Life" on the American Cancer Society webpage. His eyes lit up when he read about the Survivors Lap and he would daydream aloud about how amazing it would feel to do that "victory" lap.

A few months after we lost him, Emma and Jonah came to me and said, "We have to do Relay for Daddy."

We named our team "Arlan's Hope" because he instilled in each of us the belief that "Arlan's Hope Lives in Me."

Our family and friends have supported our effort valiantly. They have joined us walking in incredible heat and in the middle of the night to honor Arlan's fight and legacy. In 2013, I chaired our community's event and hope to do so again in the future.

We have learned that life without Arlan is diminished in some ways, yet still sweet. I notice that he is with us in the crinkle of Jonah's eyes when he smiles, in the sound of Emma's laughter and in the warmth of our embraces.

I know that we didn't do everything right, Arlan and I. Despite the best intentions to protect our children and be honest with everyone, we kept a lot of secrets from others and ourselves. Looking back, I realize that we made the best decisions we could at the time, but given the benefit of hindsight, I regret that we did not involve Emma and Jonah more. I wish I had held them out of school more, that we had stopped treatment sooner and that we had taken more time to cocoon together and just be. I do my best not to make those mistakes anymore. Although I was ill prepared for the amount of work it is being an only parent, I relish every precious moment as I see how quickly my kids are growing up.

In the time that has passed since Arlan left us, our children have blossomed. Emma is a phenomenal student who works hard and has a promising future. She has traveled internationally and become a model of community causes and service to others. As Jonah has matured, his natural sense of humor has emerged; he is one of the funniest and kindest people I know. He has also shown an incredible talent in science and math and will likely follow in his father's footsteps and become an engineer of one kind or another. I am awed by the way both children have flourished despite missing their Daddy so very much.

I sat down and began to write this memoir for several reasons, but mostly to simply try to get some of the pain out of my heart. Loving and missing Arlan is so easy, remembering his suffering at the end is a seductive trap, but I know that he was truly sick only for a short time, and pushing past that to remember him as the whole, imperfect, real and wonderful man he was is more difficult. I wanted to preserve the memories of what happened so that the details would be there for Emma and Jonah, if and when, they might want them, while I focus on memories of the whole Arlan. I also wanted to give them the gift of seeing us, their parents, through adult eyes, something I know they may not be ready to do for many years to come.

Nearly four years later, I am still haunted by much of what occurred over the eight months Arlan battled his disease. Although I initially sat down and began to write this within the first few months of his passing, it was not until more time has passed that I am able to really look at the story and undertake the painful task of examining each step of the journey. I have learned a great deal in the process. Ultimately, I am working on forgiving myself as I continue to carry the guilt of a caretaker who could not make it better and acknowledge that Arlan never expected that from me. I was the one holding on to the details, chronicling the daily fight, but Arlan moved beyond much of that. Having accepted the inevitable, Arlan was immersed in the business of making sure that the lives Emma, Jonah and I would have without him be touched by light, love and laughter.

I think that perhaps Arlan's greatest legacy is that he taught us through words and deeds that we are all one, and that love is eternal and stronger than cancer.

I still miss Arlan every day. He was, is and will be a part of me until the day I, too, leave this world. His fight taught me so much about who we were, how I want to live and what matters. His gifts to me are enduring.

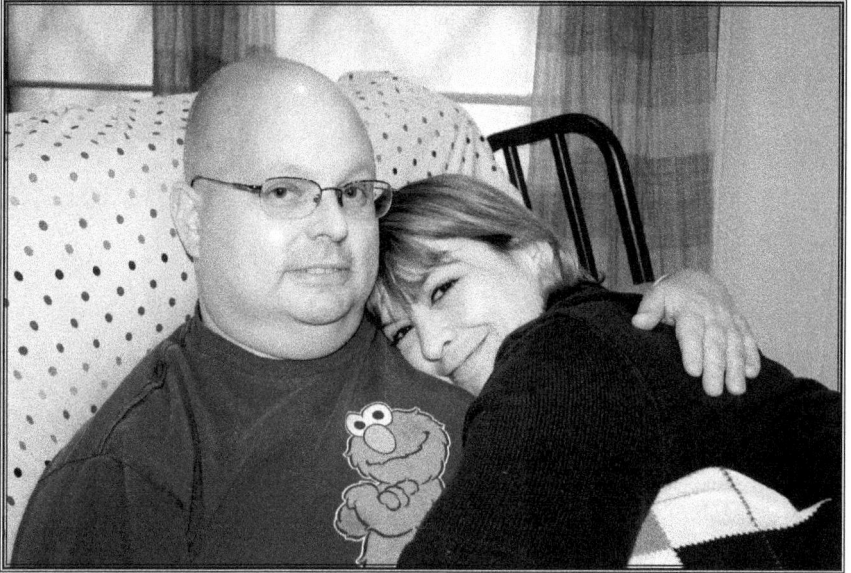

9781938842009